Holger Pettersson and Hans Ringertz

Measurements in Pediatric Radiology

With 35 Figures

Springer-Verlag
London Berlin Heidelberg New York
Paris Tokyo Hong Kong

Holger Pettersson, MD, PhD
Professor and Chairman,
Department of Radiology,
University Hospital,
S-221 Lund, Sweden

Hans Ringertz, MD, PhD
Professor and Chairman,
Department of Radiology,
Karolinska University Hospital,
S-104 Stockholm, Sweden

ISBN-13:978-1-4471-1846-6   e-ISBN-13:978-1-4471-1844-2
DOI: 10.1007/978-1-4471-1844-2

British Library Cataloguing in Publication Data
Pettersson, Holger *1942–*
   Measurements in pediatric radiology.
   1. Children.   Radiology
   I. Title   II. Ringertz, Hans *1939–*
   616.9200757
   ISBN-13:978-1-4471-1846-6

Library of Congress Cataloging-in-Publication Data
Pettersson, Holger, 1942–
   Measurements in pediatric radiology / by Holger Pettersson, Hans Ringertz.
      p.   cm.
   ISBN-13:978-1-4471-1846-6
   1. Pediatric radiology.   2. Children—Anthropometry.
I. Ringertz, Hans.   II. Title.
   [DNLM: 1. Anthropometry—in infancy & childhood.
2. Anthropometry—methods.   3. Bone Density—in infancy & childhood.
4. Radiography—in infancy & childhood.   WN 240 P485m]
RJ51.R3P48   1991
618.92′00757—dc20
DNLM/DLC
for Library of Congress   90-10455
                                                                   CIP

Typeset by Photo·graphics, Honiton, Devon

28/3830–543210 Printed on acid-free paper

Preface

A thorough knowledge of normal radiological anatomy is necessary for detection and evaluation of pathological changes. In pediatric radiology, normal anatomy and normal proportions of anatomical structures may differ considerably from the adult, and may vary during growth. Therefore, in pediatric radiology there is a multitude of measurements, that in the individual patient is important, but that for the radiologist is not meaningful or even possible to keep in mind. This holds true both for the experienced pediatric radiologist, and for those who practise pediatric radiology only occasionally. This volume is written for both categories.

In the literature, normal values are calculated and presented in many different ways, that are not always easy to compare, or easy to use in daily work. Therefore, we have revised and recalculated the data given by authors, in order to present the statistical upper and lower normal limits as between plus and minus two standard deviations (± 2SD). This means that about 2% of a normal population will be assessed as abnormally large and around 2% abnormally small with respect to the parameter assessed. In this way, the presentation throughout the book is uniform, and hopefully easy to use. All figures have been redrawn and computed in an attempt to make them as clear as possible.

A small format that can be updated has been intended in order to ensure optimal clinical use. Our purpose is only to help to differentiate between normal and abnormal, and not to make available the whole differential diagnostic list. The measurements chosen are those thought to be of most practical use in the daily routine, but in some instances methods have been included that are intended more for research applications. Generally, only one method is included for each parameter and modality, and we have tried to make the choice of methods as objective as possible. In some instances, additional methods for special cases are referred to in the "background" and/or in the reference list.

It is our sincere hope that the present volume will be of value in everyday clinical practice.

Lund and Stockholm   Holger Pettersson
January 1991   Hans Ringertz

Contents

Section 6: The Respiratory Tract

Section 7: The Cardiovascular System

Section 8: The Abdomen

Section 9: The Urinary Tract

Appendices

SECTION 1
The Skull

SK1 Width of cranial sutures in neonates and infants [radiography]

Referenced article:

Erasmie U, Ringertz H: Normal width of cranial sutures in the neonate and infant. Acta Radiol [Diagn] 1976; 17:565.

Background:

In the neonate and infant, radiologically demonstrated widening of the sutures is a generally appreciated and important sign of increased intracranial pressure. The present method is based on the lateral view, which is easy to reproduce.

Material:

Lateral skull radiographs from 64 girls and 86 boys aged 0–60 days were studied. All but 13 were considered to be mature at delivery. The lateral view of the skull was obtained with the central beam centred over the midskull. The film–focus distance was 90 cm. No correction for magnification was performed.

Method of assessment:

Both coronal sutures were assessed at levels located at approximately one-third (C1 and C2) and two-thirds (C3 and C4) of their projected course between the crown and the skull base (Figure SK1.1). In the same manner the lambdoid sutures were estimated halfway between the calvarium and the base of the skull (L1 and L2) (Figure SK1.1). The sum of these six measurements, below named the sum of suture width, was used as one of the parameters expressing the suture width (Table SK1.1). When the coronal sutures appeared V-shaped, this feature was expressed as the difference between the sums of the topnear and basal measurements of the sutures: (C1 and C2) − (C3 and C4) (Table SK1.2).

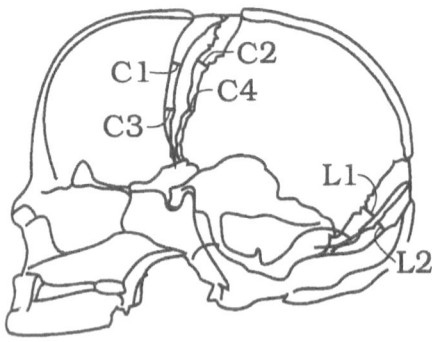

Figure SK1.1. The sites of the measurements indicated on the lateral film of a child with increased intracranial pressure. The projected course of the coronal suture is divided in three approximately equal parts and the lambdoid suture in two. (After Erasmie and Ringertz 1976.)

Table SK1.1. The upper normal value (+2SD) for the sum of suture width (C1 + C2 + C3 + C4 + L1 + L2) in neonates up to the age of 60 days. (After Erasmie and Ringertz 1976)

Upper normal value: 41mm

Table SK1.2. Upper normal value (+ 2 SD) for the V-shape (C1 + C2) − (C3 + C4) of the sutures calculated in mm related to the sum of suture width (C1 + C2 + C3 + C4 + L1 + L2) in neonates up to the age of 60 days. As an example the upper normal V-shape in an infant with a sum of suture width of 36 mm will be 4.3 mm. (After Erasmie and Ringertz 1976)

Sum of suture width (mm)	V-shape (mm)				
20	4.8	4.8	4.8	4.8	4.8
25	4.8	4.7	4.7	4.7	4.7
30	4.7	4.6	4.6	4.6	4.5
35	4.4	4.3	4.1	3.8	3.4
40	2.9	2.0	0	0	0

References:

Bützler H-O, Friedman G, Gawlich R: Plain film findings of the skull in hydrocephalus and normal infants during the first months of life. Ann Radiol 1973; 16:245.
Schuster W, Tamaela LA: Das Verhalten der Schädelnähte beim Neugeborenen und Säugling unter physiologischen und pathologischen Bedingungen. Ann Radiol 1966; 9:232.

SK2   Cranial growth/age [CT]

Referenced article:

Hahn FJ, Chu WK, Cheung JY: CT measurements of cranial growth: normal subjects. AJR 1984: 142:1253.

Background:

With CT, cranial dimensions can be obtained easily, and abnormal growth of the cranium may be detected.

Material:

CT examinations of 215 children aged 0–18 years were studied. Only patients who did not demonstrate any evidence of disease that might affect the cranial size were considered. The scans were performed in the standard supine position with an approximately 5–10° tilt from the canthomeatal line.

Method of assessment:

The midventricular section of the CT scans, showing the most prominent frontal horns of the lateral ventricles, was selected for the estimation of the cranial area, since it reflects the maximum size of the cranium. The same window setting (level 35, width 100) was used for measurements. The outer edge of the cranial vault was traced with the cursor and the enclosed cranial area was calculated, using the built-in computer program (Table SK2.1).

Table SK2.1. Normal range (−2SD to +2SD) for cranial area for infants and children up to 16 years of age. The range is given for each month up to 2 years of age and thereafter for each year. (After Hahn et al. 1984)

Age (months)	Range (cm²)	Age (months)	Range (cm²)	Age (years)	Range (cm²)
1	60– 91	13	129–158	3	148–180
2	79–109	14	131–161	4	151–189
3	90–120	15	133–163	5	154–194
4	97–128	16	135–165	6	158–197
5	103–133	17	136–166	7	163–202
6	108–139	18	137–167	8	166–205
7	113–143	19	138–168	9	168–207
8	116–145	20	140–169	10	171–210
9	118–148	21	142–171	11	172–213
10	121–151	22	143–172	12	174–215
11	124–154	23	144–174	13	176–217
12	127–156	24	145–175	14	177–218
				15	179–220
				16	181–221

SK3   Intracranial volume/age [radiography]

Referenced article:

Gordon IRS: Measurement of cranial capacity in children. Br J Radiol 1966; 39:377.

Background:

Growth patterns of the cranium measured directly as head circumference have been well documented. The present method offers a possibility of measuring the intracranial volume, using plain radiographs.

Material:

PA and lateral radiographs of the skull from 213 normal children (104 boys and 109 girls), aged 1 month – 16 years were studied. The focus–film distance was 100 cm, and no correction was made for magnification.

Method of assessment:

Internal diameters of the skull were measured according to MacKinnon et al. (Figure SK3.1). To express the volume, a modification of the MacKinnon formula was used, giving the cranial volume in cm^3 (Table SK3.1):

$$\text{Volume} = [(L \times W \times B) + (L \times W \times H)] \times 0.1594$$

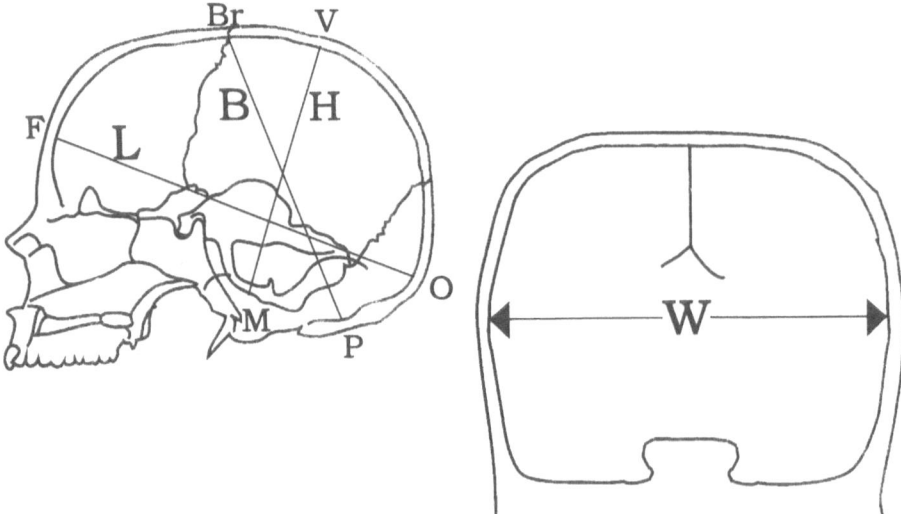

Figure SK3.1a,b Diameters measured from the internal table on the PA and lateral radiographs of the skull. L, greatest longitudinal diameter from the frontal pole (F) to the occipital pole (O); B, vertical height from the bregma (Br) to the deepest part of the posterior fossa (P); H, vertical height from the external auditory meatus (M) to the most distant point of the vertex (V); W, the greatest width at the PA projection. (After Gordon 1966.)

Table SK3.1. Normal range (−2SD to +2SD) for cranial volume according to the given formula for children from newborn to 15 years of age. Separate values for boys and girls are used. (After Gordon 1966)

Age	Volume (cm³) Boys	Volume (cm³) Girls
0 month	250–500	210–400
3 months	500–780	460–670
6 months	620–970	610–880
9 months	720–1090	720–1030
12 months	790–1190	780–1120
18 months	910–1340	840–1240
2 years	980–1440	900–1340
3 years	1080–1520	1000–1490
4 years	1130–1560	1070–1560
5 years	1180–1580	1120–1590
6 years	1210–1610	1150–1600
7 years	1230–1630	1170–1610
8 years	1250–1650	1180–1610
9 years	1270–1670	1190–1610
10 years	1290–1690	1200–1610
11 years	1310–1710	1210–1610
12 years	1330–1730	1220–1610
13 years	1350–1750	1220–1610
14 years	1370–1770	1230–1610
15 years	1390–1790	1230–1610

References:

Cronqvist S: Roentgenologic evaluation of cranial size in children. A new index. Acta Radiol [Diagn] 1978; 7:97.

McCammon RW: Human growth and development. Thomas; Springfield, Illinois, 1970.

Nellhaus G: Head circumference from birth to eighteen years. Pediatrics 1968; 41:106.

Pryor HB: Charts of normal body measurements and revised width–weight table in graphic form. J Pediatr 1966; 68:615.

SK4 Volume of sella turcica/age [radiography]
Volume of sella turcica/height [radiography]

Referenced article:

Underwood LE, Radcliffe WB, Guinto FC: New standards for the assessment of sella turcica volume in children. Radiology 1976; 119:651.

Background:

The sellar volume may be important in the evaluation of a short child. If it is found to be small, this might serve as a stimulus for prompt and thorough evaluation of pituitary function.

Material:

Conventional PA and lateral radiographs of the skull from 38 normal children were studied.

Method of assessment:

For calculation of the volume (Table SK4.1), the following formula was used:

Volume $V = 0.5 \times (L \times D \times W)$ (Figure SK4.1)

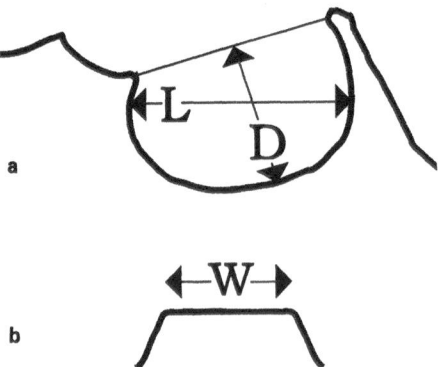

Figure SK4.1. Lateral projection of the sella (**a**) and frontal projection of the sellar floor (**b**), showing the diameters measured: L, the longest AP diameter; D, the longest perpendicular dimension between the diaphragmatic line and the sellar floor; W, the width of the sellar floor. (After Underwood et al. 1976.)

Table SK4.1. Normal range (−2 SD to + 2 SD) for sellar volume related to age from 1 to 16 years and related to body height from 70 to 170 cm. (The normal range for individuals older than 16 years or taller than 170 cm is 271–923 mm³). (After Underwood et al. 1976)

Age (years)	Range (mm³)	Body height (cm)	Range (mm³)
1	100–335	70	75–313
2	156–506	80	116–410
3	164–536	90	156–506
4	173–566	100	171–558
5	181–596	110	185–610
6	189–625	120	199–662
7	197–655	130	214–715
8	205–685	140	228–767
9	214–715	150	242–819
10	222–744	160	257–871
11	230–774	170	271–923
12	238–804		
13	246–834		
14	255–863		
15	263–893		
16	271–923		

References:

Chilton LA, Dorst JP, Garn SM: The volume of the sella turcica in children: new standards. AJR 1983; 140:797.

Di Chiro G, Nelson KB: The volume of the sella turcica. AJR 1962; 87:989.

Silverman FN: Roentgen standards for size of the pituitary fossa from infancy through adolescence. AJR 1957; 78:451.

SK5   Interorbital distance/age [radiography]

Referenced article:

Hansman CF: Growth of interorbital distance and skull thickness as observed in roentgenographic measurements. Radiology 1966; 86:87.

Background:

The interorbital distance and its changes with age are of interest in several types of skeletal dysplasia.

Material:

Radiographs from sinus examinations of 5351 healthy children (2652 boys and 2699 girls), aged 0–15 years were studied. The sinus films were taken on an angle board with nose and forehead touching the cassette and the X-ray tube in the vertical position. The focus–film distance was 28 inches (71 cm). No correction was made for magnification.

Method of assessment:

Using a caliper, the shortest distance between the orbits was measured (Table SK5.1).

Table SK5.1. Normal range (−2SD to +2SD) for the interorbital distance in boys and girls aged 1–15 years. (After Hansman 1966)

Age (years)	Interorbital distance (mm)	
	Boys	Girls
1	13.7–21.5	13.4–21.2
2	14.2–22.4	14.5–21.8
3	15.2–23.0	15.1–22.6
4	15.9–24.1	15.9–23.5
5	16.4–25.0	17.1–24.1
6	17.1–26.0	17.7–25.0
7	17.6–26.9	18.2–25.7
8	18.3–27.3	18.7–26.2
9	18.9–28.0	19.2–26.9
10	19.3–29.0	19.6–27.5
11	20.4–29.5	20.2–28.2
12	21.0–29.9	20.6–28.8
13	21.6–30.3	21.1–29.4
14	22.0–31.1	21.5–29.6
15	22.8–31.7	21.7–29.8

SK6 Length of the hard palate in the newborn [radiography]

Referenced article:

Austin JHM, Preger L, Siris E, Taybi H: Short hard palate in newborn: roentgen sign of mongolism. Radiology 1969; 92:775.

Background:

Shortening of the hard palate is a sign of Down's syndrome. However, today, more accurate, non-radiological methods are available for the diagnosis of Down's syndrome.

Material:

Lateral skull radiographs from 182 normal newborns were examined.

Method of assessment:

The length of the hard palate, from the anterior maxillary process to the posterior termination of the bony hard palate was measured on the film (Figure SK6.1; Table 6.1).

Table SK6.1. Normal range (−2SD to +2SD) for the length from the anterior maxillary process to the posterior termination of the bony hard palate. (After Austin et al. 1969)

	Range (mm)
Preterm newborns	26.2–32.8
Term newborns	28.2–34.5

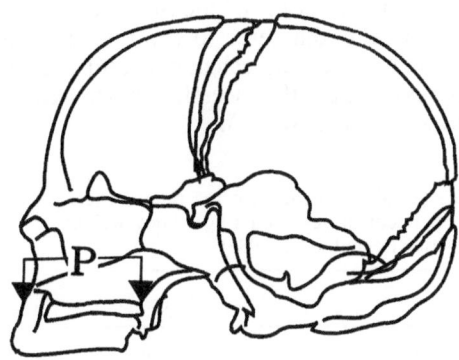

Figure SK6.1. The length (P) of the hard palate is measured from the anterior maxillary process to the posterior edge of the bony hard palate (between *arrows*). (After Austin et al. 1969.)

SK7 Ventricular size at birth ratios [ultrasound]

Referenced article:

Poland RL, Slovis TL, Shankaran S: Normal values for ventricular size as determined by real time sonographic techniques. Pediatr Radiol 1985; 15:12.

Background:

Real time sector ultrasonography is today the primary routine method for evaluation of intracranial contents of neonates.

Material:

Seventy-three real time sector scans of infants of 28–48 weeks' gestational age, with no evidence of intracranial disease were studied.

Method of measurement:

In the coronal plane, the distance between the lateral superior aspect of the frontal horns (ventricular diameter) at the level of the head of the caudate nuclei was measured as was the distance between the inner tables of the skull (brain diameter) at this level (Figure SK7.1a). Similar readings were obtained at the level of the midglomus of the choroid plexus in the ventricular atria. If the outermost margin of the ventricle was not seen, then the outer edge of the choroid plexus was used instead.

In the parasagittal planes, the frontal horns of the lateral ventricles were identified and the thickness of parenchyma extending from the anterior wall of the frontal horn to the frontal bone was measured (frontal mantle) (Figure SK7.1b). Similarly, in the same plane, the occipital horn (if identified) was used to obtain the thickness of the occipital cortex (occipital mantle). In most cases the latter measure was not obtainable. Both frontal and occipital cortical thicknesses were taken as the largest distance from the tip of the horn to the bone in an arc of 90° from the point of measurement.

The ratio of the ventricular diameter to the thickness of brain diameter at each level in the coronal plane was calculated and the ratio of the occipital cortical mantle thickness (when the occipital horn was seen) to the frontal cortical mantle thickness (Table SK7.1).

Table SK7.1 Normal range (−2SD to +2SD) for the ratios. These ratios were constant, independent of gestational age, body weight or head circumference. (After Poland et al. 1985)

Ratio	Range
Occipital/frontal mantle (OM/FM)	0.49–1.07
Ventricles/brain at caudate (IV/TC)	0.23–0.42
Ventricles/brain at atria (IV/TC)	0.40–0.60

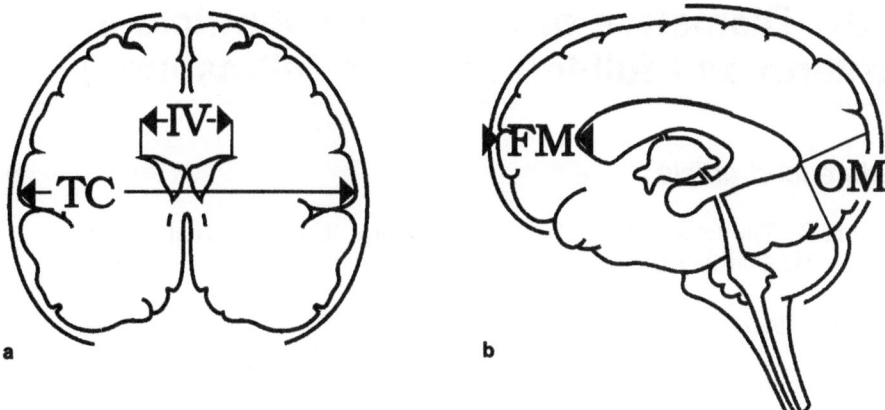

a   b

Figure SK7.1. a Measures in the coronal plane at the level of the head of the caudate nucleus. TC, transcalvarial distance (brain diameter); IV, intraventricular distance (ventricular diameter). **b** Measures in the sagittal plane. FM, distance from the anterior wall of the frontal horn to the frontal bone (frontal mantle); OM, greatest distance from the posterior portion of the occipital horn to the occipital bone within a 90° sector (occipital mantle). (After Poland et al. 1985.)

SK8 Diameters of the lateral ventricle in preterm and full-term infants [ultrasound]

Referenced article:

Virkola K: The lateral ventricle in early infancy. Thesis, Helsinki, 1988 (ISBN: 952–90012–9–0).

Background:

See subsection SK7.

Material:

A total of 81 normal, full-term infants and 112 very low birth weight preterm (< 1500 g) infants were followed with ultrasound examinations from birth to 9 months of age.

Method of assessment:

Using a sector scanner the following measurements were obtained.

Axial measures: ventricular midbody and brain hemisphere width (Figure SK8.1a).

Coronal measures: combined coronal width of both ventricular bodies (Figure SK8.1b).

The normal ranges for full-term and very low weight preterm normal infants are shown in Tables SK8.1 and SK8.2, respectively.

Table SK8.1. Healthy full-term infants. Normal ranges (−2SD to +2SD) for different ultrasonographic measurements of the neonatal and infant brain. Values are given for each month of age up to 9 months. (After Virkola 1988)

Age (months)	Midbody thickness (mm)	Hemispheric width (mm)	Coronal ventricular width (mm)
0	11.5–14.1	39.0–46.4	21.6–27.9
1	11.9–14.8	40.6–48.2	22.4–29.0
2	12.3–15.4	42.1–50.0	23.2–30.1
3	12.7–16.1	43.7–51.9	24.0–31.1
4	13.1–16.7	45.2–53.7	24.8–32.2
5	13.5–17.3	46.8–55.6	25.6–33.3
6	13.9–18.0	48.3–57.4	26.4–34.3
7	14.3–18.6	49.8–59.2	27.1–35.4
8	14.7–19.3	51.4–61.1	27.9–36.5
9	15.1–19.9	52.9–62.9	28.7–37.5

14

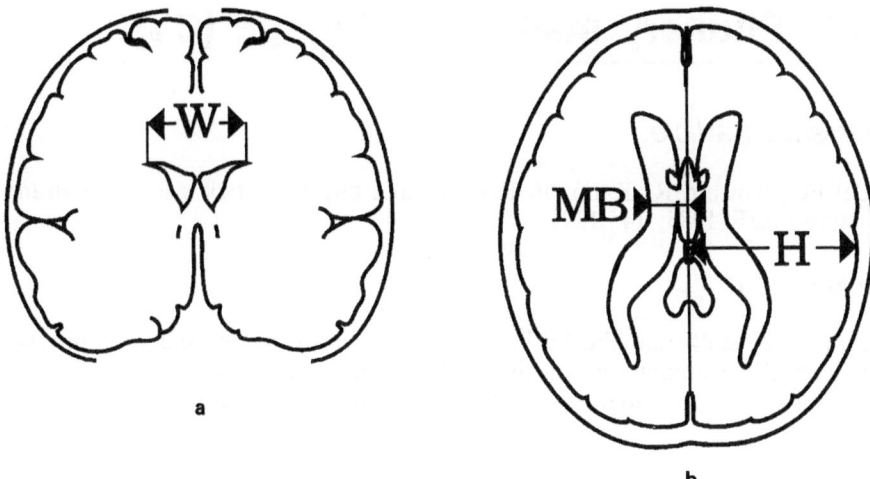

Figure SK8.1. a Axial measures of ventricular midbody width (MB) and brain hemisphere width (H). **b** Coronal measure of combined coronal ventricular width (W). MB, midline to midbody lateral wall distance; H, midline to calvarium distance; W, coronal width of both ventricular bodies. (After Virkola 1988.)

Table SK8.2. Very low birth weight preterm normal infants. Normal ranges (−2SD to +2SD) for different ultrasonographic measurements of the neonatal and infant brain. Values are given for each month of age up to 9 months. (After Virkola 1988)

Age (months)	Midbody thickness (mm)	Hemispheric width (mm)	Coronal ventricular width (mm)
−3	7.0–11.3	23.6–34.0	15.5–23.9
−2	7.7–12.1	25.9–36.4	16.6–25.6
−1	8.3–12.9	28.3–38.9	17.8–27.2
0	8.9–13.8	30.7–41.3	18.9–28.9
1	9.5–14.6	33.1–43.8	20.0–30.5
2	10.1–15.5	35.5–46.2	21.1–32.2
3	10.7–16.3	37.9–48.7	22.2–33.8
4	11.3–17.2	40.3–51.1	23.3–35.5
5	11.9–18.0	42.7–53.6	24.4–37.1
6	12.5–18.8	45.0–56.0	25.6–38.8
7	13.1–19.7	47.4–58.5	26.7–40.5

Table SK8.3 Normal range of ventricular index (−2SD to +2SD). This index is the same in all normal neonates and infants, including the very low birth weight group. (After Virkola 1988)

Normal range	0.27–0.36

15

SK9   Pituitary stalk diameter/age [CT]

Referenced article:

Seidel FG, Towbin R, Kaufman RA: Normal pituitary stalk size in children: CT study. AJR 1985; 145:1297.

Background:

The pituitary stalk and the basilar artery are easily recognised on contrast-enhanced CT examinations of the skull. In children, early detection of an abnormal stalk is essential in endocrine and neoplastic disease.

Material:

A total of 659 normal CT scans, in children aged newborn–18 years (53% boys and 47% girls) were studied. The CT examinations were performed using a 9.6 s scanning time in the dynamic scanning mode with table incrementation. The scans were begun during bolus injection of 2 ml/kg Hypaque Meglumine 60%. The slice thickness was 10 mm in most cases, but comparison with 5 mm scans showed no significant difference.

Table SK9.1. Normal range (−2SD to +2SD) for the pituitary stalk diameter in boys and girls up to the age of 15 years. (After Seidel et al. 1985)

Age (years)	Diameter (mm)	
	Boys	Girls
0–0.5	1.3–2.5	1.2–2.5
0.5–1.0	1.3–2.5	1.2–2.6
1	1.3–2.6	1.2–2.6
2	1.3–2.6	1.3–2.7
3	1.3–2.7	1.3–2.8
4	1.4–2.8	1.3–2.9
5	1.4–2.9	1.3–3.0
6	1.4–2.9	1.3–3.0
7	1.4–3.0	1.4–3.1
8	1.4–3.1	1.4–3.2
9	1.5–3.2	1.4–3.3
10	1.5–3.2	1.4–3.4
11	1.5–3.3	1.4–3.5
12	1.5–3.4	1.5–3.6
13	1.5–3.5	1.5–3.7
14	1.6–3.5	1.5–3.7
15	1.6–3.6	1.5–3.8

Method of assessment:

The measures were performed at sections through the midstalk, with window 80–150 HU, level 40 HU, using a micrometer. The diameter of the pituitary stalk (PS) (Table SK9.1) and the basilar artery (BS) was measured, and the ratio PS/BS was calculated (Table SK9.2).

Table SK9.2. Normal range (−2SD to +2SD) for the ratio between the diameter of the pituitary stalk and diameter of the basilar artery in boys and girls 0–15 years of age. (After Seidel et al. 1985)

Boys	0.35–0.80
Girls	0.39–0.90

Reference:

Peyster RG, Hoover ED, Adler LP: CT of the normal pituitary stalk. AJNR 1984; 5:45.

SECTION 2
The Spine

SP1 Transverse diameter of foramen occipitale magnum/age [radiography]

Referenced article:

Bliesener JA, Schmidt LR: Normal and pathological growth of the foramen magnum shown in the plain radiograph. Pediatr Radiol 1980; 10:65.

Background:

The size of the foramen occipitale magnum may be of interest as children with Arnold–Chiari malformation have an increased diameter irrespective of whether or not there is a concomitant hydrocephalus. However, the diagnostic value of the measurement is probably limited.

Material:

Skull radiographs of 36 children aged 0–2.1 years and 128 children aged 2.1–14 years old were studied. The radiographs were obtained with the central beam in a 30–40° craniocaudal incident angle (semiaxial). The film–focus distance was 100 cm. The magnification factor was not corrected for.

Method of assessment:

The maximum width of the foramen occipitale was measured (Figure SP1.1; Table SP1.1).

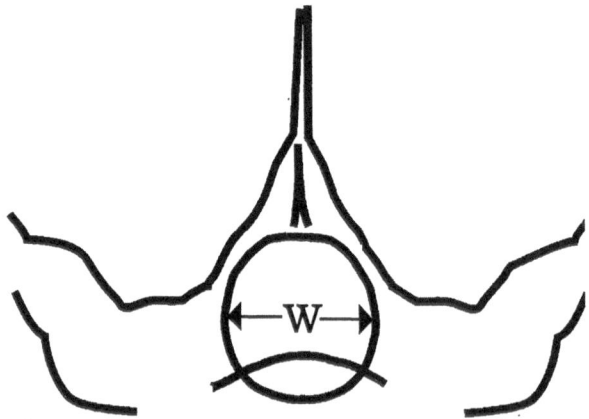

Figure SP1.1. The maximal width (W) of the foramen magnum, as measured in the semiaxial projection. (After Bliesener and Schmidt 1980.)

Table SP1.1. Normal average maximum width of the foramen occipitale magnum for children below 2.1 years of age. Normal range (−2SD to +2SD) above 2.1 years. (After Bliesener and Schmidt 1980)

Age (Years)	—	+3 months	+6 months	+9 months
0	20.0	21.7	23.3	25.0
1	26.7	28.3	30.0	31.7
2	33.3			
2.1–14	30.5–39.0			

References

Coin DG, Malkasian DR: Foramen magnum. In: Newton TH, Potts DG (eds) Radiology of the skull and brain, vol 1, book 1. CV Mosby, St Louis, 1971, p. 275.

Krogness KG, Nyland H: Posterior fossa measurements. II. Size of the posterior fossa in myelomeningocele. Pediatr Radiol 1978; 6:193.

McRae DL: Craniovertebral junction. In: Newton TH, Potts DG (eds) Radiology of the skull and brain, chapter 14. CV Mosby, St Louis, 1971, p. 260.

SP2 Sagittal diameter of cervical spinal canal/age, [radiography]
Sagittal diameter of cervical spinal canal/height [radiography]

Referenced article:

Markuske H: Sagittal diameter measurements of the bony cervical spinal canal in children: Pediatr Radiol 1977; 6:129.

Background:

The sagittal diameter of the cervical spinal canal may be important in the evaluation of a possible intraspinal mass occupying lesion. Most authors measuring the sagittal diameter state that, regardless of age, the diameter either gradually decreases from C1 to C7 or diminishes from C1 to C3 and remains unchanged between C4 and C7. Yousefzadeh et al. (1982), however, pointed out that at ages below 11 years a slight widening of the lower cervical canal might exist in up to 30% of normal individuals. Therefore, the sagittal diameter is an uncertain measure for evaluation of possible intraspinal processes. However, it is valuable for assessing conditions that may lead to spinal stenosis. The present article was chosen as it is based on the largest amount of 'normal' material (Tables SP2.1 and SP2.2).

Table SP2.1. Normal range (−2SD to +2SD) of the sagittal diameter of the bony cervical spinal canal according to age and sex. Above the age of 6 years, sex differences were < 0.1 mm and deviations between boys and girls are therefore not given. (After Markuske 1977)

	Sagittal diameter (mm)				
	3–6 years			7–10 years Range	11–14 years Range
	Range	Deviation			
Cervical level		Boys	Girls		
C1	17.3–22.5	+0.3	−0.3	18.0–23.2	18.5–24.1
C2	15.3–20.5	+0.3	−0.3	16.8–20.8	17.2–21.6
C3	13.4–18.6	+0.3	−0.2	15.2–19.2	15.8–19.8
C4	13.2–18.4	+0.2	−0.2	15.1–18.7	15.5–19.1
C5	13.1–18.3	+0.2	−0.2	14.9–18.5	15.2–18.8
C6	13.2–18.0	+0.2	−0.3	14.6–18.2	14.9–18.5
C7	13.1–17.5	+0.3	−0.3	14.2–17.8	14.4–18.0

Material:

Lateral radiographs of 120 normal children, aged 3–14 years were studied. Focus–film distance was 150 cm, and magnification was not corrected for.

Table SP2.2. Average sagittal diameter of the bony cervical spinal canal (mm), according to body height. Stabilised variation not available. (After Markuske 1977)

Cervical level	Height (cm)							
	91–100	101–110	111–120	121–130	131–140	141–150	151–160	161–170
C1	19.0	19.9	20.6	20.5	20.7	21.2	21.3	21.4
C2	17.2	17.7	18.5	18.8	18.9	19.2	19.5	19.6
C3	15.3	15.9	16.8	17.2	17.3	17.6	17.8	17.9
C4	15.0	15.6	16.5	16.9	17.0	17.2	17.2	17.5
C5	14.9	15.5	16.4	16.6	16.7	16.9	17.1	17.2
C6	14.8	15.4	16.1	16.4	16.4	16.6	16.8	16.9
C7	14.6	15.3	15.7	16.0	16.1	16.0	16.5	16.4

Methods of assessment:

The sagittal diameter of the spinal canal was measured from the middle of the posterior surface of the vertebral body to the nearest point of the ventral line of the cortex seen at the junction of the spinal processes and laminae (Figure SP2.1).

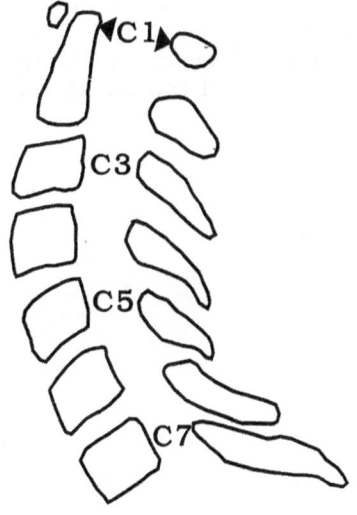

Figure SP2.1. Sagittal diameter of the bony spinal canal, defined as the distance between the middle of the posterior surface of the vertebral body to the nearest point on the ventral line of the cortex at the junction of the spinous processes and laminae. (After Markuske 1977.)

References:

Boijsen E: The cervical spinal canal in intraspinal expansive processes. Acta Radiol 1954; 42:101.
Hinck VC, Hopkins CE, Savara BS: Sagittal diameter of the cervical spine in children. Radiology 1962; 79:97.
Payne EE, Spillane DJ: The cervical spine. An anatomico-pathological study of 70 specimens (using a special technique) with particular reference to the problem of cervical spondylosis. Brain 1957; 80:571.
Yousefzadeh DK, El-Khoury GY and Smith WL: Normal sagittal diameter and variation in the pediatric cervical spine. Radiology 1982; 144:139.

SP3 Sagittal diameter of the cervical spinal canal in infants [radiography]

Referenced article:

Naik DR: Cervical spinal canal in normal infants. Clin Radiol 1970; 21:323.

Background:

See subsection SP2.

Material:

Twenty-five lateral radiographs of the cervical spine in 25 normal post-mortem infants were compared with measurements at autopsy. The radiographs were taken at a film–focus distance of 90 cm, and no correction was made for magnification.

Method of measurement:

In infancy, the anterior margin of the spinal process is impossible to define as it is still cartilaginous. However, Naik showed that in infants the height of the spinal process at its base is equal to its sagittal thickness, and hence the internal sagittal diameter may be calculated as shown in Figure SP3.1 and the normal range determined (Table SP3.1).

Table SP3.1. Normal range (−2SD to +2SD) for sagittal diameter of the cervical spinal canal in infants. Ranges are given for each vertebral level. (After Naik 1970)

Vertebral level	Normal range (mm)
C2	9.9–15.0
C3	8.2–14.8
C4	8.7–14.6
C5	9.6–14.8
C6	10.0–15.2
C7	8.6–15.9

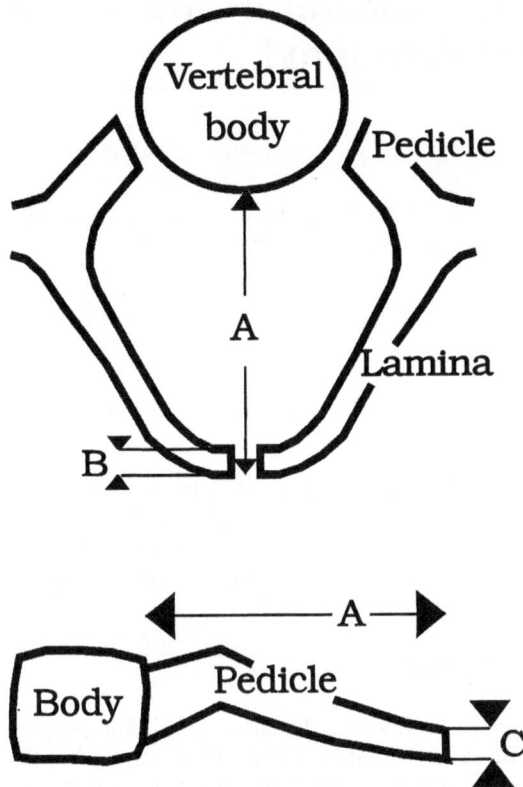

Figure SP3.1. Method for measuring the sagittal diameter. A, Distance between posterior border of vertebral body to the tip of the spinous process. B, Thickness of the spinous process. C, Height of the spinous process. In infants B = C, and therefore the sagittal diameter of the spinal canal can be calculated from the lateral projection: sagittal diameter = A − C. (After Naik 1970.)

SP4   Sagittal diameter of the lumbar spinal canal/age [radiography]

Referenced article:

Hinck VC, Hopkins CE, Clark WM: Sagittal diameter of the lumbar spinal canal in children and adults. Radiology 1965; 85:929.

Background:

See subsection SP2.

Material:

Lateral lumbar spine radiographs of 209 patients, aged 3 years and above were studied. All subjects with significant anomalies and other problems likely to influence growth and development were eliminated from the review. The radiographic examinations were performed with a film–focus distance of 90 cm, and magnification was not corrected for.

Method of assessment:

The sagittal diameter was defined as the shortest midline perpendicular distance from the vertebral body to the inner surface of the neural arch. Normal ranges of sagittal diameter for ages between 3 and 15 years are given in Table SP4.1.

Table SP4.1. Normal range (−2SD to +2SD) of sagittal diameter of the lumbar spinal canal for ages between 3 and 15 years and both sexes. The range is given for all lumbar segments. (After Hinck et al. 1965)

Age (years)	Sagittal diameter, range (mm)				
	L1	L2	L3	L4	L5
3	16.1–22.6	16.4–21.4	15.2–20.0	15.4–20.0	15.1–20.9
4	16.2–22.8	16.4–21.6	15.3–20.3	15.5–20.5	15.1–21.4
5	16.3–23.0	16.5–21.9	15.4–20.7	15.5–21.0	15.0–21.9
6	16.4–23.2	16.5–22.1	15.5–21.1	15.5–21.5	15.0–22.4
7	16.6–23.5	16.6–22.4	15.6–21.5	15.5–22.0	15.0–22.9
8	16.7–23.7	16.6–22.6	15.7–21.8	15.5–22.5	15.0–23.4
9	16.8–23.9	16.7–22.9	15.8–22.2	15.6–22.9	15.0–23.8
10	16.9–24.1	16.7–23.1	15.9–22.6	15.6–23.4	14.9–24.3
11	17.1–24.4	16.8–23.4	16.0–22.9	15.6–23.9	14.9–24.8
12	17.2–24.6	16.8–23.6	16.2–23.3	15.6–24.4	14.9–25.3
13	17.3–24.8	16.9–23.9	16.3–23.7	15.7–24.9	14.9–25.8
14	17.5–25.0	16.9–24.1	16.4–24.0	15.7–25.4	14.9–26.3
15	17.6–25.3	17.0–24.4	16.5–24.4	15.7–25.9	14.8–26.8

SP5 Interpeduncular distance/age [radiography]

Referenced article:

Hinck VC, Clark, Jr WM, Hopkins CE: Normal interpediculate distances (minimum and maximum) in children and adults. AJR 1966; 97:141.

Background:

Measurements of the interpeduncular distance may be of value for evaluation of mass-occupying lesions in the vertebral column, as well as for evaluation of skeletal dysplasias. As was said for the sagittal measurements, most authors have not accounted for different magnification factors. This is important, as modern radiographic techniques may use a greater magnification than those used in studies published in the 1960s and earlier.

Material:

Radiographs from 353 children under the age of 19 years were studied. An attempt was made to eliminate subjects with significant anomalies and problems likely to influence growth and development. A film–focus distance of 90 cm was used, and no correction was made for magnification.

Method of assessment:

The interpeduncular distance was defined as the shortest distance between the medial surfaces of the pedicles of a given vertebra. Normal ranges are given for interpedunculate distances for cervical, thoracic and lumbar spine (Table SP5.1).

Reference:

Schwartz GS: Width of spinal canal in growing vertebrae with special reference to sacrum: maximum interpediculate distances in adult and children. AJR Rad Ther Nucl Med 1956; 76:476.

Table SP5.1. Normal range (−2SD to +2SD) for interpeduncular distance (mm), according to age

	Age (years)												
	3	4	5	6	7	8	9	10	11	12	13	14	15
Cervical spine													
C3	21-28.	21-28	21-28	22-29	22-29	22-29	22-29	23-30	23-30	23-30	23-30	23-31	24-31
C4	22-29	22-29	22-29	22-29	23-30	23-30	23-30	23-30	24-31	24-31	24-31	24-31	25-32
C5	22-29	22-29	22-30	23-30	23-30	23-30	23-31	24-31	24-31	24-32	24-32	25-32	25-32
C6	22-30	22-30	22-30	22-30	23-31	23-31	23-31	23-31	24-31	24-32	24-32	24-32	24-32
C7	21-29	21-29	21-29	21-30	21-30	22-30	22-30	22-30	22-30	22-31	23-31	23-31	23-31
Thoracic spine[a]													
T1	18-26	18-26	18-26	18-26	19-26	19-26	19-26	19-27	19-27	19-27	19-27	19-27	20-27
T2	15-22	15-22	15-22	15-23	16-23	16-23	16-23	16-23	16-23	16-23	16-23	16-23	16-24
T3	14-20	14-20	15-20	15-20	15-20	15-21	15-21	15-21	15-21	15-21	15-21	15-21	16-21
T4	14-19	14-19	14-19	14-19	14-19	14-20	14-20	14-20	14-20	15-20	15-20	15-20	15-21
T5	13-19	13-19	14-19	14-19	14-19	14-19	14-19	14-20	14-20	14-20	14-20	15-20	15-20
T6	13-19	13-19	13-19	13-19	14-19	14-19	14-19	14-20	14-20	14-20	14-20	14-20	14-20
T7	13-19	13-19	13-19	14-20	14-20	14-20	14-20	14-20	14-20	14-20	14-20	14-20	14-20
T8	13-19	14-20	14-20	14-20	14-20	14-20	14-20	14-20	14-20	14-20	15-21	15-21	14-20
T9	14-20	14-20	14-20	14-20	14-20	14-20	14-20	14-21	14-21	15-21	15-21	15-21	15-21
T10	14-20	14-20	14-20	14-20	14-20	14-21	14-21	14-21	14-21	15-21	15-21	15-21	15-21
T11	14-21	14-22	15-22	15-22	15-22	15-22	15-22	15-23	15-23	16-23	16-23	16-23	16-23
T12	16-24	17-24	17-24	17-24	17-24	17-25	18-25	18-25	18-25	18-25	18-26	19-26	19-26
Lumbar spine[a]													
L1	17-24	17-25	17-25	18-25	18-25	18-26	19-26	19-26	19-27	19-27	20-27	20-27	20-28
L2	17-24	17-25	18-25	18-25	18-25	18-26	19-26	19-26	19-26	20-27	20-27	20-27	20-27
L3	17-25	18-25	18-26	18-26	18-26	19-26	19-27	19-27	19-27	20-27	20-28	20-28	21-28
L4	17-27	17-27	18-28	18-28	18-28	18-29	19-29	19-29	19-30	20-30	20-30	20-31	21-31
L5	19-31	19-31	20-32	20-32	20-32	21-33	21-33	22-33	22-34	22-34	22-35	23-35	23-35

[a] After Hinck et al. (1966).

SP6   Size of vertebral body and intervertebral disc/age [radiography]

Referenced article:

Brandner MF: Normal values of the vertebral body and intervertebral disk index during growth. AJR 1970; 10:618.

Background:

The vertebral growth takes place both by enchondral ossification in the vertical direction and periosteal ossification in the horizontal direction. Measurements of vertical and sagittal vertebral body diameters permit comparative studies of enchondral and periosteal growth, and in different types of skeletal dysplasias this might enhance recognition of pathological features of the vertebrae.

Material:

A total of 187 radiographs of thoracic and lumbar spines from newborns up to adolescents were studied. Careful attention was paid to exclude children with virtual vertebral diseases or degenerative syndromes. Traumatic lesions of the spine were included if they were outside the studied region.

The film–focus distance was 110 cm, and the magnification factor was 1.13–1.25. This magnification was not corrected for, as indices were used.

Table SP6.2. Intervertebral disc index (I_D, the minimal intervertebral space/maximal vertical diameter of the vertebra below). Normal range (−2SD to +2SD) is given for selected vertebral segments for each year of age up to 15 years. The index is given for both sexes as no significant sex difference has been shown. (After Brandner 1970)

Age	T11–12/T12	T12–LI/LI	L1–L2/L2	L2–L3/L3
0	0.20–0.49	0.19–0.46	0.21–0.44	0.18–0.53
1	0.17–0.43	0.17–0.41	0.18–0.40	0.16–0.47
2	0.15–0.41	0.16–0.39	0.17–0.39	0.16–0.45
3	0.14–0.39	0.15–0.38	0.16–0.38	0.15–0.43
4	0.13–0.37	0.14–0.36	0.15–0.37	0.15–0.42
5	0.13–0.36	0.14–0.35	0.15–0.37	0.15–0.41
6	0.12–0.35	0.13–0.34	0.14–0.36	0.14–0.39
7	0.11–0.33	0.13–0.33	0.13–0.35	0.14–0.38
8	0.11–0.32	0.12–0.32	0.13–0.35	0.14–0.37
9	0.10–0.31	0.12–0.32	0.12–0.34	0.14–0.36
10	0.10–0.30	0.12–0.31	0.12–0.34	0.14–0.36
11	0.09–0.29	0.11–0.30	0.11–0.33	0.13–0.35
12	0.09–0.29	0.11–0.29	0.11–0.33	0.13–0.34
13	0.08–0.28	0.11–0.29	0.11–0.32	0.13–0.33
14	0.08–0.27	0.10–0.28	0.10–0.32	0.13–0.32
15	0.08–0.26	0.10–0.27	0.10–0.31	0.13–0.32

Method of assessment:

Measurements were performed according to Figure SP6.1. The central beam was projected through the first lumbar vertebra. Using these measurements, the following indices were calculated:

Vertebral body index $= I_{VB} = V/S$ (Table SP6.1).

where

$V =$ the largest vertical measurements of the body

$S =$ the sagittal anteroposterior diameter in the smallest anteroposterior measurement of the body.

Intervertebral disc index $= I_D = D/V$ (Table SP6.2)
where
$D =$ intervertebral disc thickness.

Table SP6.1. Vertebral body index (I_{VB}, vertical/sagittal anteroposterior diameter) for some vertebral bodies according to age. Normal ranges ($-2SD$ to $+2SD$) are given separately for the sexes when significant differences were observed. (After Brandner 1970)

	Age (years)						
				4–12		> 13	
	Newborn	0–1.5	1.5–3	Girls	Boys	Girls	Boys
T12	0.69–0.93	0.75–1.06	0.73–0.79	0.74–0.98	0.67–0.88	0.64–1.23	0.60–1.07
L1	0.76–0.99	0.87–1.09	0.73–1.05	0.73–1.00	0.70–0.90	0.88–1.22	0.74–0.99
L2	0.80–1.04	0.83–1.19	0.79–1.03	0.67–0.97		0.84–1.22	0.70–1.05
L3	0.81–1.08	0.81–1.15	0.72–1.04	0.67–0.91		0.80–1.20	0.68–1.03

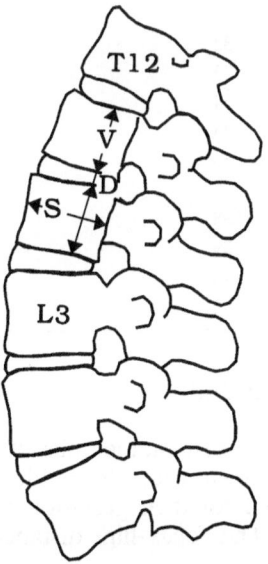

Figure SP6.1. Method for measurement of vertebral bodies and disc spaces. V, vertical vertebral diameter; S, sagittal anteroposterior vertebral diameter; D, minimal intervertebral disc thickness.

SP7   Spinal length at birth/gestational age [radiography]

Referenced article:

Kuhns LR, Holt JF: Measurement of thoracic spine length on chest radiographs of newborn infants. Radiology 1975; 116:395.

Background:

Measurement of spinal length has been used to determine intrauterine fetal size and crown–rump length to assess embryological age. Thoracic spine length increases linearly with increasing gestational age between 26 and 41 weeks (Table SP7.1). It is closely correlated to total spine length, but relatively unaffected by birth weight. Thoracic spine length is probably a more accurate means of assessing trunk length than the crown–rump measurements.

Table SP7.1. Normal range (−2SD to +SD) of thoracic spinal length (T1–T12), according to gestational age at birth. (After Kuhns et al. 1975)

Gestational age (weeks)	Range (mm)
25	47–67
26	50–70
27	52–72
28	55–75
29	57–77
30	60–80
31	62–82
32	65–85
33	68–88
34	70–90
35	73–93
36	75–95
37	78–98
38	80–100
39	83–103
40	85–105
41	88–108

Material:

AP chest radiographs of 88 newborn infants of 26–41 weeks' gestational age were studied. The children had a weight, length and head circumference within 2SD for their gestational age.

The focus–film distance was 102 cm, and magnification was not corrected for.

Method of assessment:

The distance from the superior edge of the first thoracic vertebral body to the inferior edge of the twelfth thoracic vertebral body was measured.

SP8 Thoracic kyphosis/age [radiography]

Referenced article:

Fon GT, Pitt MJ, Cole Thies A, Jr: Thoracic kyphosis: range in normal subjects. AJR 1979; 134:979.

Background:

Some degree of thoracic convexity in the sagittal plane is normal, whereas an increased thoracic curvature (thoracic kyphosis) is common in several conditions, such as Scheurmann's disease, congenital spinal anomalies, metabolic and neurological disturbances, and inflammatory and traumatic conditions. Measurements of the kyphosis facilitates definition of the pathological state, and follow-up examinations during treatment.

Material:

Chest radiographs in the lateral projection from 54 children and adolescents, aged 2–19 years were studied. The individuals had no signs or symptoms of any abnormality of the heart, lungs, or thoracic skeleton.

The examinations were made with the patients standing, with a focus–film distance of 1.8 m, and with the patient's arms lifted above the shoulders. Normal ranges of thoracic kyphosis in children aged between 5 and 15 years are given in Table SP8.1.

Table SP8.1. Normal range (−2SD to +2SD) for thoracic kyphosis in children between 5 and 15 years of age when standing with the arms raised. (After Fon et al. 1979)

Age (years)	Range of thoracic kyphosis (degrees)	
	Boys	Girls
5	7.6–38.0	5.1–36.7
6	7.8–38.2	5.5–37.1
7	8.0–38.4	5.8–37.4
8	8.2–38.6	6.2–37.8
9	8.4–38.8	6.5–38.1
10	8.6–39.0	6.9–38.5
11	8.8–39.2	7.2–38.8
12	9.0–39.4	7.5–39.1
13	9.3–39.7	7.9–39.5
14	9.5–39.9	8.2–39.8
15	9.7–40.1	8.6–40.2

Method of measurement:

The degree of kyphosis was measured by a modification of the Cobb technique, according to Figure SP8.1.

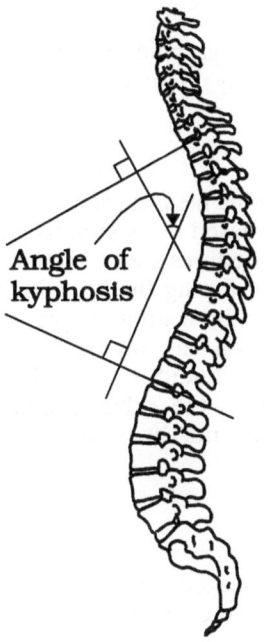

Angle of
kyphosis

Figure SP8.1. Method for measurement of kyphosis. (After Fon et al. 1979.)

Reference:

Cobb RJ: Outline for the study of scoliosis. Am Acad Orthop Surg 1948; 5:261.

SP9 Diameter of the spinal cord [conventional myelography]

Referenced article:

Boltshauser E, Hoare RD: Radiographic measurements of the normal spinal cord in childhood. Neuroradiology 1976; 10:235–237.

Background:

Only a few reports on radiographic measurements of the spinal cord in children are documented, and most are based on post-mortem studies. Absolute values obtained after myelographic procedures are of limited value, as the magnification pattern may differ considerably during the examination. Therefore, the ratio of the spinal cord width to the subarachnoid space width has been considered. The present article is based on air myelography. It should be noticed that replacement of the subarachnoid fluid with air severely disturbs the hydrodynamic equilibrium within the subarachnoid space. Thus the values found for air myelography may not be valid for myelography with water-soluble contrast media.

Material:

Air myelograms of 110 children aged 1 month to 15 years were studied. The myelograms were normal, and the children did not suffer from conditions which might influence the size of the spinal cord or subarachnoid space.

Method of assessment:

The spinal cord and the subarachnoid space were measured in the sagittal diameter at the midvertebral level, at right angles to the long axis of the cord, and in the transverse diameter at interpedicular level. The ratio between the diameter of the cord and the subarachnoid space was calculated for each level (Tables SP9.1 and SP9.2). The ratios did not differ with respect to age or sex.

Table SP9.1. Normal range (−2SD to +2SD) for sagittal spinal cord/subarachnoid space ratio in children up to the age of 15 years. (After Boltshauser and Hoare 1976)

C1	0.44–0.68	T1	0.39–0.63	T7	0.41–0.73
C2	0.47–0.67	T2	0.38–0.66	T8	0.40–0.72
C3	0.51–0.71	T3	0.39–0.67	T9	0.41–0.69
C4	0.51–0.71	T4	0.37–0.69	T10	0.42–0.70
C5	0.49–0.69	T5	0.35–0.71	T11	0.44–0.68
C6	0.46–0.70	T6	0.38–0.70	T12	0.44–0.68
C7	0.43–0.67				

Table SP9.2 Normal range (−2SD to +2SD) for transverse spinal cord/subarachnoid space ratio in children up to the age of 15 years. (After Boltshauser and Hoare 1976)

T5	0.52–0.80	T8	0.51–0.79	T10	0.52–0.76
T6	0.55–0.79	T9	0.51–0.79	T11	0.50–0.78
T7	0.53–0.77			T12	0.43–0.76

References:

DiChiro G, Fisher RL: Contrast radiography of the spinal cord. Arch Neurol 1964; 11:125.
Nordqvist L: The sagittal diameter of the spinal cord and subarachnoid space in different age groups. A roentgenographic post-mortem study. Acta Radiol 1964; Suppl 227.

SP10   Diameter of the spinal cord
[CT and myelography]

Referenced article:

Pettersson H, Harwood-Nash CDF: CT and myelography of the spine and cord. Techniques, anatomy and pathology in children. Springer-Verlag; Berlin, Heidelberg, New York, 1982, pp. 33.

Background:

Using water-soluble contrast media, the hydrodynamic equilibrium of the subarachnoid space is not disturbed as it is during an air myelography. Using CT examination, exact measurements can be achieved (Table SP10.1).

Table SP10.1. Ranges of normal cord diameters (mm) at different levels and ages at CT contrast myelography. (After Pettersson and Harwood-Nash 1982)

Level	Age				
	0 < 6 months	6 months < 2 years	2 < 6 years	6 < 12 years	12 < 18 years
C3					
AP	4.5–5.5	6.5–8.0	6.0–7.5	7.0–8.0	6.5–8.0
Lat.	6.0–7.0	8.5–10.5	9.5–11.0	9.5–11.5	11.0–13.5
C7–T1					
AP	4.5–5.5	5.5–6.5	5.0–7.0	5.5–6.0	6.0–6.5
Lat.	5.5–6.5	7.5–9.0	6.5–11.0	7.5–9.5	8.0–9.5
T6					
AP	3.0–3.5	4.5–5.5	4.5–6.0	5.0–6.0	5.5–6.0
Lat.	3.0–3.5	5.0–7.0	5.5–8.0	6.5–8.0	7.5–8.0
Conus					
AP	4.0–4.5	5.5–7.0	6.5–7.5	7.0–8.5	7.0–9.0
Lat.	4.5–5.5	6.5–9.0	8.0–9.0	9.0–9.5	8.0–11.0

Material:

The CT myelograms of 45 children aged 0–18 years were studied. The CT myelograms were normal, and the patients had no disease that might change the size of the cord.

Method of assessment:

To avoid influences on the measurement values caused by CT window levels and width, the window level was set as the mean between the attenuation values for the contrast medium within the subarachnoid space and for the cord (Seibert et al. 1981). The measurements were performed with a narrow window width (20–40 Hounsfield units).

References:

Resjö IM, Harwood-Nash DC, Fitz CR, Chuang S: Normal cord in infants and children examined with computed tomographic metrizamide myelography. Radiology 1979; 130:691.
Seibert CE, Barnes JE, Dreisbach JN, Swanson WB, Heck RJ: Accurate CT measurement of the spinal cord using metrizamide: physical factors. AJNR 1981; 2:75.

SECTION 3
Pelvis and Hips

PH1 Iliac angle and iliac index/age [radiography]

Referenced article:

Caffey J, Ross S: Pelvic bones in infantile mongoloidism. AJR 1958; 80:458

Background:

Measurement of the acetabular angle may be of value in evaluation of skeletal dysplasias, and also a means of following the acetabular ossification in congenital dislocation of the hip. The iliac angle and iliac index may be used to diagnose Down's syndrome – even if more accurate cytogenetic methods are available today.

Material:

AP radiographs of 500 unselected newborn infants (Table PH1.1) were studied. The central beam was directed about 2 cm above the symphysis.

Table PH1.1. Normal ranges (−2SD to +2SD) of acetabular and iliac angles as well as iliac index in degrees for neonates and infants. The corresponding range in Down's syndrome is given in parentheses. (After Caffey and Ross 1958)

	Age			
	0–3 months		3–12 months	
	Normal	(Down)	Normal	(Down)
Acetabular angle	18–37	(7–25)	14–28	(3–19)
Iliac angle	44–66	(30–56)	43–72	(29–55)
Iliac index	65–97	(49–80)	60–96	(29–67)

Method of assessment:

The acetabular angle is defined as the angle between a line drawn through the Y-cartilages and a line connecting the most craniolateral point of the bony acetabulum and its most caudomedial point on the ilium (Figure PH1.1). The iliac angle is defined as the angle between the line through the Y-cartilages, and a line drawn through the most lateral point of the iliac body and the most lateral point of the iliac wing (Figure PH1.1).

The iliac index is the sum of both acetabular angles and both iliac angles divided by 2.

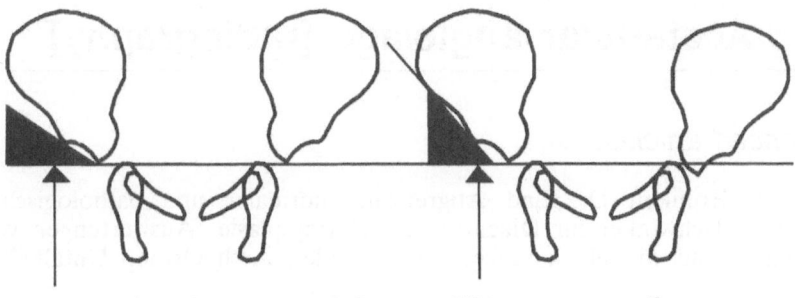

Acetabular angle   **Iliac angle**

Figure PH1.1. Definition of acetabular and iliac angles. (After Caffey and Ross 1958.)

PH2   Acetabular angle/age [radiography]

Referenced articles:

Tönnis D, Brunken D: Eine Abgrenzung normaler und pathologischer Hüftpfannendachwinkel zur Diagnose der Hüftdysplasie. Auswertungen von 2294 Pfannendachwinkeln kindlicher Hüftgelenke. Arch Orthop Unfall-Chir 1968; 64:197.

Caffey J, Ames R, Silverman WA, Ryder CT, Hough G: Contradiction of congenital dysplasia – predislocation hypothesis of congenital dislocation of hip through study of normal variation in acetabular angles at successive periods in infancy. Pediatrics 1956; 17:632.

Table PH2.1. Normal range (−2SD to +2SD) for the acetabular angle in girls and boys for the right and left hip expressed in degrees. The angle is related to age in months up to the age of 6 years (72 months). (After Tönnis and Brunken 1968; Caffey et al. 1956)

Age (months)	Acetabular angle			
	Girls		Boys	
	Right hip	Left hip	Right hip	Left hip
0	18.3–38.1	19.5–39.8	16.0–33.4	17.6–35.4
1	16.9–35.9	18.0–37.7	14.6–31.9	16.3–33.8
2	16.3–35.0	17.4–36.8	14.0–31.2	15.8–33.1
3	15.8–34.4	16.9–36.2	13.6–30.7	15.4–32.6
4	15.4–33.8	16.5–35.6	13.2–30.3	15.0–32.2
5	15.0–33.3	16.2–35.1	12.9–30.0	14.7–31.8
6	14.7–32.8	15.8–34.6	12.6–29.6	14.4–31.5
7	14.4–32.4	15.5–34.2	12.3–29.3	14.2–31.1
8	14.2–32.0	15.3–33.8	12.0–29.1	13.9–30.8
9	13.9–31.6	15.0–33.5	11.8–28.8	13.7–30.6
10	13.7–31.2	14.8–33.1	11.6–28.5	13.5–30.3
11	13.5–30.9	14.5–32.8	11.3–28.3	13.3–30.1
12	13.2–30.6	14.3–32.5	11.1–28.1	13.1–29.8
18	12.1–28.9	13.1–30.8	10.0–26.9	12.1–28.6
24	11.1–27.5	12.1–29.5	9.1–25.9	11.2–27.5
30	10.3–26.2	11.3–28.2	8.3–25.0	10.5–26.6
36	9.5–25.1	10.5–27.1	7.6–24.2	9.8–25.7
42	8.8–24.0	9.8–26.1	6.9–23.4	9.2–24.9
48	8.1–23.0	9.1–25.2	6.3–22.8	8.6–24.2
54	7.5–22.1	8.5–24.3	5.7–22.1	8.0–23.5
60	6.9–21.3	7.9–23.4	5.1–21.5	7.5–22.9
66	6.4–20.4	7.3–22.6	4.6–20.9	7.0–22.3
72	5.8–19.7	6.7–21.9	4.1–20.4	6.5–21.7

Background:

The acetabular angle (Table PH2.1), as well as the iliac angle and iliac index, are important means for detection of skeletal dysplasia, and for evaluation of congenital dislocation of the hip. Much interest has also been given to the value of these angles for the diagnosis of Down's syndrome, but this has less impact today, given modern genetic techniques.

Material:

Assessments were made on AP radiographs of the pelvis, obtained in 719 girls and 428 boys, aged 0–7 years (Tönnis and Brunken 1968) and AP radiographs of 500 unselected newborn infants (Caffey et al. 1956).

Method of assessment:

The acetabular angle was defined as the angle between the transverse line through the cartilages of the ilium and a line connecting the medial and lateral ends of the bony edge of the acetabulum (Figure PH1.1).

Reference:

Lönnerholm T, Almberg B: Hip joint stability after the neonatal period. 1. Value of measuring the acetabular angle. Acta Radiol 1979; 20:200.

PH3 Acetabular coverage of the femoral head/age [radiography]

Referenced article:

Eklöf O, Ringertz H, Samuelsson L: The percentage of migration as indicator of femoral head position. Acta Radiol [Diagn] 1988; 29:363.

Background:

Subluxation of the femoral head caused by, for instance, neurological disturbances may be difficult to define. The present method gives a simple means of defining lateral migration of the femoral head relative to the acetabulum.

Material:

Radiographs from examination of the abdomen or the pelvis of 507 children (255 boys and 252 girls), aged 0.25–11.67 (mean: 6.7) years were studied. None of the children had any history, or clinical or radiological findings raising suspicion of neuromuscular, significant spinal or hip disease.

Methods of assessment:

On the AP film of the hip in neutral position, a line (Hilgenreiner's horizontal) is drawn at the level of the Y-cartilages connecting the innermost parts of the iliac bones (Figure PH3.1). Perpendiculars to this horizontal are drawn through the acetabular edge (Perkin's line) and tangential to the medial and lateral outlines of the femoral head. The migration is defined as the linear part of the femoral head which is located lateral to Perkin's line. This fraction is expressed as a percentage of the whole width of the femoral head.

The percentage migration was determined for both hips in the 507 cases reviewed. A computerized analysis was carried out establishing the upper 98 percentile (+ 2SD) of the normal variations for this material (Table PH3.1).

Table PH3.1. Upper normal values of femoral head migration (98th percentile) for different age groups. The differences between sides are included. (After Eklöf et al. 1988)

	Age (years)			
	< 4	> 4 < 8	> 8 < 12	> 12
Upper normal migration	16%	19%	22%	24%
Upper normal difference between sides in all age groups: 12%				

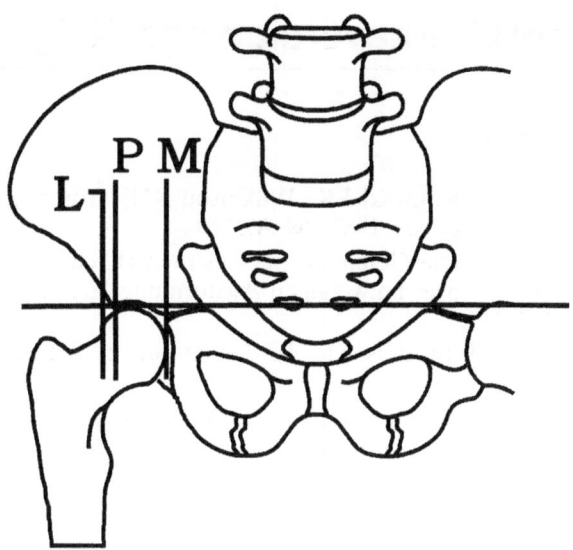

Figure PH3.1. Lines drawn to calculate acetabular coverage (lateral migration) of the femoral head. Perkin's line (P) through the acetabular edge, and lines tangential to the medial (M) and lateral (L) outlines of the femoral head are drawn perpendicular to Hilgenreiner's horizontal. (After Eklöf et al. 1988.)

PH4 Femoral anteversion/age [CT]

Referenced articles:

Murphy SB, Simon SR, Kijewski PK, Wilkinson RH, Griscom NT: Femoral anteversion. J Bone Joint Surg 1987; 69-A:1169.

Von Lantz T, Mayet A: Die Gelenkkörper des menschlichen Hüftgelenkes in der progredierten Phase ihrer umweigigen Ausformung. Z Anat Entwicklungsgeschichte 1953; 117:317.

Fabry G, MacEwen GD, Strands AR, Jr: Torsion of the femur. J Bone Joint Surg 1973; 55-A:1726.

Dunlop K, Strands AR, Jr, Hollister LC, Jr, Gaul JS, Jr, Streit HA: A new method for determination of torsion of the femur. J Bone Joint Surg 1953; 35-A:289.

Background:

There are a number of published methods for measurement of the anteversion of the femoral neck, based on radiography, fluoroscopy and CT. The three-dimensional anatomy of the hip is complicated, and the large number of methods may indicate that the ideal method has still to be found.

The radiographic methods are based on radiographs with the central beam directed parallel to the long axis of the femur, or on a combination of AP and lateral projections through the pelvis. All methods give a high radiation dose to the pelvis.

CT examination provides possibilities for measurement of the angle with a lower radiation dose and should, therefore, be used today. The method described below has been shown to correlate well with direct anatomical measurements.

Table PH4.1. Normal range (−2SD to +2SD) for femoral neck anteversion in neonates and infants from the 28th week of gestation to 60 months of age as measured from specimens. (After Von Lantz and Mayet 1953)

Age	Femoral anteversion (degrees)
28 weeks	2–47
32 weeks	10–53
36 weeks	15–55
40 weeks	17–55
6 months	18–54
12 months	19–53
24 months	18–50
36 months	17–46
48 months	16–41
60 months	15–38

Method of measurement (Murphy et al. 1987)*:*

The patient is examined supine, with the long axis of the femur parallel to the long axis of the scanner. Transaxial CT sections are taken, and the angle of anteversion is defined as described in Figure PH4.1.

No series of normal values has so far been published for CT evaluation of the anteversion angle. Generally, the degree of anteversion is subject to great individual variation. The values given in Table PH4.1 were obtained from an anatomical study of 242 specimens (Von Lantz and Mayet 1953), while those given in Table PH4.2 are based on the Dunlop method applied on 864 children (Fabry et al. 1973).

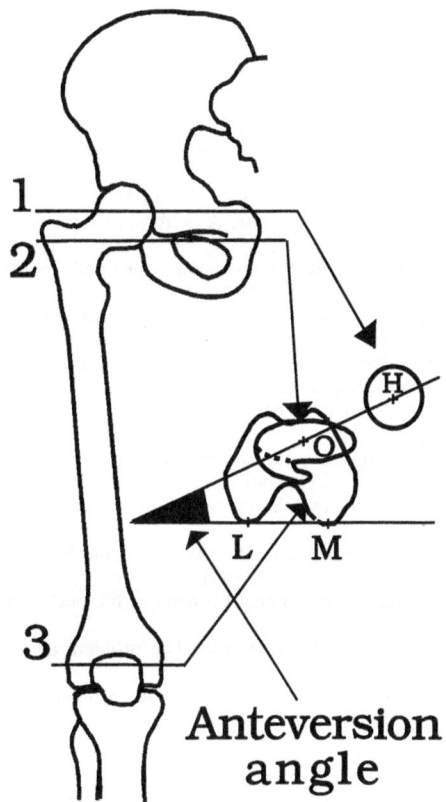

Figure PH4.1. CT assessment of the anteversion angle. Three CT sections are used:

1. One image defines the location of the centre of the femoral head (H)
2. The second image defines the centre of the base of the femoral neck, as the centroid of a cross-section of the femur at the base of the femoral neck, (O)
3. The third image defines the plane of the condylar axis, defined by the line tangential to the most posterior aspect of the lateral (L) and medial (M) condyle

The three sections are superimposed. The angle of anteversion is then the angle between the line HO and the line ML (After Murphy et al. 1987.)

Table PH4.2. Normal range (−2SD to +2SD) for femoral neck anteversion for children of both sexes between 1 and 15 years of age. (After Fabry et al. 1973)

Age (years)	Femoral anteversion (degrees)	Age (years)	Femoral anteversion (degrees)	Age (years)	Femoral anteversion (degrees)
1	15.1–45.8	6	10.4–40.1	11	5.7–34.5
2	14.1–44.7	7	9.5–39.0	12	4.8–33.3
3	13.2–43.5	8	8.5–37.9	13	3.8–32.2
4	12.3–42.4	9	7.6–36.7	14	2.9–31.1
5	11.3–41.3	10	6.6–35.6	15	2.0–29.9

References:

Billing L: Roentgen examination of the proximal femur end in children and adolescents. A standardized technique also suitable for determination of the collum-, anteversion-, and epiphyseal angles. A study of slipped epiphysis and coxa plana. Acta Radiol 1954; Suppl 110.

Dunlop K, Strands AR, Jr, Hollister LC, Jr, Gaul JS, Jr, Streit HA: A new method for determination of torsion of the femur. J Bone Joint Surg 1953; 35-A:289–311.

Dunn DM: Anteversion of the neck of the femur. A method of measurement. J Bone Joint Surg 1952; 34-B:181–186.

Edholm P: Nomogram for measuring the anteversion angle and angulation of fracture from roentgenograms. Acta Radiol 1972; 12:856–864.

Egund N, Palmer J: Femoral anatomy described in cylindrical coordinates using computed tomography. Acta Radiol [Diagn] 1984; 25:209.

Henriksson L: Measurement of femoral neck anteversion and inclination. A radiographic study in children. Acta Orthop Scand [Suppl] 1980; 186.

Hernandez RJ, Tachdjian MO, Poznanski AK, Dias LS: CT determination of femoral torsion. AJR 1981; 137:97–101.

Magilligan DJ: Calculation of the angle of anteversion by means of horizontal lateral roentgenography. J Bone Joint Surg 1956; 38-A:1231–1246.

Norman O: Röntgenologisk bestämning av collumanteversionsvinklar och dess praktiska tillämpning (in Swedish). Nord Med 1966; 75:318.

Ogata K, Goldsand EM: A simple biplanar method of measuring femoral anteversion and neck-shaft angle. J Bone Joint Surg 1979; 61-A:846–851.

Rogers SP: A method for determining the angle of torsion of the neck of the femur. J Bone Joint Surg 1931; 13:821–824.

Ryder CT, Crane L: Measuring femoral anteversion. The problem and a method. J Bone Joint Surg 1953; 35-A:321–328.

Weiner DS, Cook AJ, Hoyt WA, Jr, Oravec CE: Computed tomography in the measurement of femoral anteversion. Orthopedics 1978; 1:299–306.

PH5 Shaft/neck angle of the femur/age [radiography]

Referenced articles:

Von Lantz T, Mayet A: Die Gelenkkörper des menschlichen Hüftgelenkes in der progredierten Phase ihrer umweigigen Ausformung. Z Anat Entwicklungsgeschichte 1953; 117:317.

Bogdanov G: A method of determining the true angle of deviation in a fracture. Br J Radiol 1950; 23:497.

Background:

As with femoral anteversion, many measurement methods have been proposed to define the femoral shaft/neck angle. Several of these do not take into consideration the anteversion, measure directly on the AP film, and give a considerable error. In one method which combines fluoroscopy and radiography the leg is rotated to a true AP of the plane through the femoral shaft/neck angle in the fluoroscope, and then an AP radiograph is obtained. The most accurate method is that described by Bogdanov (1950), using one AP and one lateral projection, but this means a high radiation dose.

Normal values: as with the anteversion angle, the femoral shaft/neck angle (Figure PH5.1) is also subject to large individual variations. The values given (Table PH5.1) were obtained in an anatomical study (Von Lantz and Mayet 1953).

Table PH5.1. Normal range (−2SD to +2SD) for the shaft/neck angle of the femur. Angles in degrees are given for different ages for boys and girls together. (After Von Lantz and Mayet 1953)

Age	Shaft/neck angle	Age	Shaft/neck angle
28 gw[a]	113–141	6 years	122–149
32 gw	111–140	7 years	122–149
36 gw	113–141	8 years	122–149
40 gw	119–143	9 years	122–149
6 months	120–145	10 years	122–149
1 year	120–147	11 years	122–149
2 years	121–148	12 years	122–149
3 years	121–148	13 years	122–149
4 years	121–148	14 years	121–148
5 years	122–149	15 years	121–148

[a] gw: gestation weeks

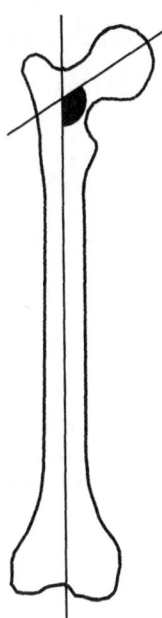

Figure PH5.1. Femoral shaft/neck angle.

References:

Hamacher G: Röntgenologische Normalwerte des Hüftgelenkes, CCD-Winkel und AT-Winkel. Orthop Prax 1974; H.1/X:23.

Tönnis D: Normal values of the hip joint for the evaluation of X-rays in children and adults. Clin Orthop 1976; 119:39.

Zippel H: Untersuchungen zur Normalentwicklung der Formelemente am Hüftgelenk im Wachstumsalter. Beitr Orthop 1971; 18:H5:225.

PH6 Appearance and size of femoral head/age [radiography]

Referenced article:

Pettersson H, Theander G: Ossification of femoral head in infancy. I. Normal standards. Acta Radiol [Diagn] 1979: 20:170.

Background:

In skeletal dysplasias and congenital hip disease, not only is the osseous development of the acetabulum influenced, but also that of the femoral head. Therefore, the age at appearance of the ossification centre, as well as the size of the centre according to age, should be observed.

Material:

AP films of the abdomen or pelvis of 455 infants, aged 0–12 months were studied. Children with disease or trauma of the hip were excluded.

Method of assessment:

The maximum height of the ossification centre, perpendicular to the growth plate, was measured using a magnifying glass (Table PH6.1).

Table PH6.1. Normal range (−2SD to +2SD) (mm) of the height of the ossification centre of the femoral head in infants aged between 1 and 12 months, as calculated for both sexes. Girls are on the average 0.4 mm above the mean, whereas boys are 0.4 mm below. (After Pettersson and Theander 1979)

Age (months)	Range (mm)	Age (months)	Range (mm)	Age (months)	Range (mm)
1	0.0–5.1	2	0.0–5.8	3	0.0–6.6
4	0.1–7.3	5	0.9–8.0	6	1.6–8.7
7	2.3–9.4	8	3.0–10.1	9	3.7–10.8
10	4.4–11.5	11	5.1–12.2	12	5.8–12.9

Table PH6.2. The statistical probability of having one or two ossified femoral head centres at different ages (months) for the two sexes. (After Pettersson and Theander 1979)

Age	Probability (%)	
	Boys	Girls
0	0.7	0.4
1	2.0	1.6
2	5.7	6.0
3	14.9	20.3
4	33.8	50.2
5	59.9	80.1
6	81.3	94.1
7	92.7	98.4
8	97.4	99.6
9	99.1	99.9
10	99.7	100.0
11	99.9	100.0
12	100.0	100.0

PH7 Angle measurements of the hip in infants [ultrasound]

Referenced articles:

Graf R: Fundamentals of sonographic diagnosis of infant hip dysplasia. J Pediatr Orthop 1984; 4:735.

Zieger M, Schultz RD: Ultrasonography of the infant hip. Part III: clinical application. Pediatr Radiol 1987; 17:226.

Background:

Ultrasound is today the method of choiced for early detection of dysplasia and dislocation of the neonatal and infant hip, and also for definition of the severity of disease, as well as for monitoring the progress of healing. The examination may be performed as a dynamic study during provocation manoeuvres, or as a more static morphological examination, based on evaluation of the anatomy of the hip joint. For such evaluation, the present angles are used.

Material:

A sample of 600 normal infants, aged 0–6 months was studied. The examinations were performed with the children in the lateral position, the transducer being placed on the greater trochanter.

Method of assessment:

The angles alpha, beta, and delta were measured as described in Figure PH7.1. Normal ranges are given in Table PH7.1.

Table PH7.1 Normal ranges (−2SD to +2SD) for the three angles alpha, beta, and delta of the neonatal and infant hip as determined by ultrasound. The angles are expressed in degrees and related to the age in months for each half month of age. (After Zieger and Schultz 1987)

Age (months)	Alpha range (degrees)	Beta range (degrees)	Delta range (degrees)
0.0	54.2–67.2	47.8–68.0	65.1–80.9
0.5	56.4–67.8	44.7–73.0	68.0–81.7
1.0	57.3–68.1	43.5–75.0	69.1–82.1
1.5	57.9–68.3	42.5–76.6	70.0–82.4
2.0	58.5–68.5	41.7–77.9	70.8–82.6
2.5	59.0–68.6	41.0–79.1	71.5–82.8
3.0	59.5–68.7	40.3–80.2	72.1–83.0
3.5	59.9–68.9	39.7–81.2	72.6–83.2
4.0	60.3–69.0	39.2–82.1	73.1–83.4
4.5	60.6–69.1	38.6–82.9	73.6–83.5
5.0	61.0–69.2	38.1–83.7	74.1–83.7
5.5	61.3–69.3	37.7–84.5	74.5–83.8
6.0	61.6–69.4	37.2–85.2	74.9–83.9

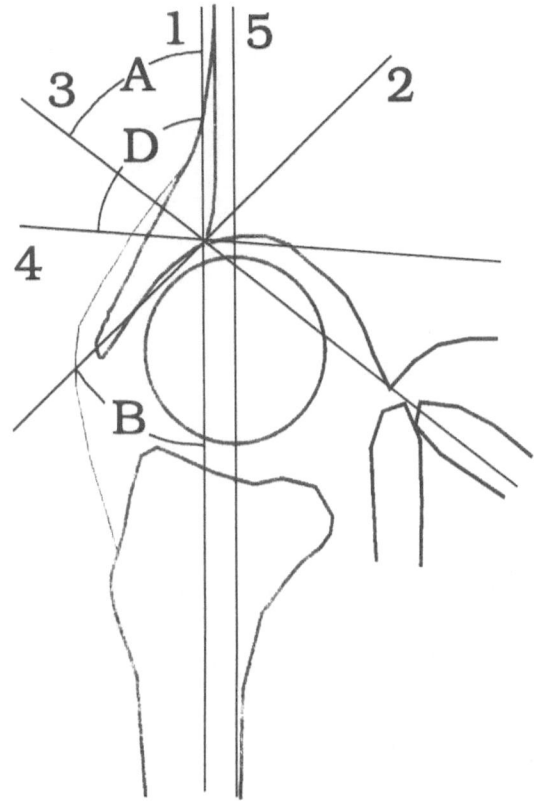

Figure PH7.1. Lines and angles used for sonographic evaluation of the infant hip.

1. The baseline paralleling the os ilium proximal to the acetabular rim along the basis of the gluteus minimus muscle.
2. The inclination line following the labrum, beginning at its base at the acetabular rim.
3. The acetabular roof line, connecting the acetabular rim with the Y-cartilage in the acetabular fossa.
4. The concavity line parallel to the osseous part of the acetabular roof in the proximity of the rim.

The angles are defined as follows:

Alpha (acetabular roof angle): the angle between the baseline (1) and the acetabular roof line (3).

Beta (inclination angle): the angle between the base line (1) and the inclination line (2).

Delta (the concavity angle): the angle between the baseline (1) and the concavity line (4).

(After Graf 1984; Zieger and Schultz 1987.)

SECTION 4
The Extremities

EX1 Carpal length [radiography]

Referenced article:

Poznanski AK, Hernandez RJ, Guire KE, Bereza UL, Garn SM: Carpal length in children – a useful measurement in the diagnosis of rheumatoid arthritis and some congenital malformation syndromes. Radiology 1978; 129:661.

Background:

Shortening of the carpal length occurs in juvenile chronic arthritis and in several malformation syndromes, but it may be difficult to determine and to quantify. The present method is suitable for children and is independent of age and skeletal maturation.

Material:

A sample comprising 539 radiographs of healthy children (280 boys, 259 girls), aged 1.5–15.4 years was studied.

Method of assessment:

The measure RM (Figure EX1.1) is a line from a point on the third metacarpal to the midgrowth plate of the radius. The point on the metacarpal is defined as the intersection of the central axis of this bone with the proximal end. The midportion of the distal radius growth plate can be determined by simple visual observation.

The measure M2 (Figure EX1.1) is defined as the maximum length of the second metacarpals.

The measure W (Figure EX1.1) was determined as the line joining the most radial point on the base of the second metacarpal and the most ulnar point on the base of the fifth metacarpal. When the bases of these bones were curved the midpoint of the lateral curvature was used.

The relationships W versus RM and M2 versus RM were calculated (Tables EX1.1 and EX1.2).

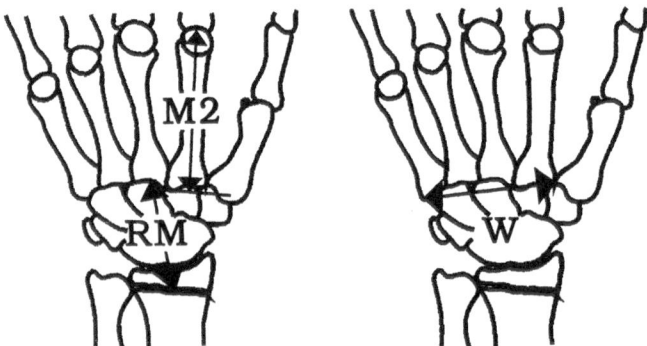

Figure EX1.1. Measurements for evaluation of carpal length. The lines RM, M2 and W are defined in the text. (After Poznanski et al. 1978.)

Table EX1.1. Normal range (−2SD to +2SD) for the radiometacarpal length (RM) (mm) related to the intermetacarpal width (W) for boys and girls. A normal girl with an intermetacarpal width of 36 mm has a 96% probability of having a radiometacarpal length between 32 and 38 mm. (After Poznanski et al. 1978)

Intermetacarpal width, W (mm)	+0	+1	+2	+3	+4	+5	+6	+7	+8	+9
Boys										
20	19-26	20-27	21-28	22-29	23-30	23-30	24-31	25-32	26-33	27-34
30	27-35	28-35	29-36	30-37	31-38	31-39	32-39	33-40	34-41	35-42
40	36-43	36-44	37-44	38-45	39-46	40-47	40-48	41-48	42-49	43-50
Girls										
20	20-26	21-27	21-27	22-28	23-29	24-30	24-30	25-31	26-32	27-33
30	27-33	28-34	29-35	30-36	30-36	31-37	32-38	33-39	33-39	34-40
40	35-41	36-42	36-42	37-43	38-44	39-45	39-45	40-46	41-47	42-48

Table EX1.2. Normal range (-2SD to +2SD) (mm) for the radiometacarpal length (RM) related to the length of the second metacarpal (M2). As an example, a normal boy with the length of his second metacarpal 72 mm has a 96% probability of having a radiometacarpal length between 39 and 47 mm. (After Poznianski et al. 1978)

Metacarpal length, M2 (mm)	+0	+1	+2	+3	+4	+5	+6	+7	+8	+9
Boys										
20	18–26	18–26	19–26	19–27	19–27	20–28	20–28	21–28	21–29	22–29
30	22–30	22–30	23–30	23–31	24–31	24–32	24–32	25–32	25–33	26–33
40	26–34	26–34	27–35	27–35	28–35	28–36	28–36	29–37	29–37	30–37
50	30–38	30–38	31–39	31–39	32–39	32–40	32–40	33–41	33–41	34–41
60	34–42	34–42	35–43	35–43	36–43	37–44	37–44	37–45	37–45	38–45
70	38–46	39–46	39–47	39–47	40–47	41–48	41–48	41–49	41–49	42–50
80	42–50	43–50	43–51	43–51	44–52	44–52	45–52	45–53	45–53	46–54
Girls										
20	18–24	18–25	18–25	19–25	19–26	20–26	20–26	20–27	21–27	21–27
30	21–28	22–28	22–29	22–29	23–29	23–30	23–30	24–30	24–31	24–31
40	25–31	25–32	25–32	26–32	26–33	26–33	27–33	27–34	28–34	28–34
50	28–35	29–35	29–35	29–36	30–36	30–37	30–37	31–37	31–38	31–38
60	32–38	32–39	32–39	33–39	33–40	33–40	34–40	34–41	34–41	35–41
70	35–42	36–42	36–42	36–43	37–43	37–43	37–44	38–44	38–45	38–45
80	39–45	39–46	39–46	40–46	40–47	40–47	41–47	41–48	41–48	42–48

EX2 Carpal angle/age [radiography]

Referenced article:

Poznanski AK, Garn SM, Shaw HA: The carpal angle in congenital malformation syndromes. Ann Radiol 1976; 19:141–150.

Background:

Variations in the carpal angle occur in several congenital malformations. The normal values of this angle vary with age, race and sex.

Material:

PA radiographs of the hands in neutral position in 455 normal children (251 boys and 204 girls) were studied.

Method of assessment:

The angle between the tangent to the proximal edge of the lunate and scaphoid and the tangent to the proximal edge of the lunate and the triquetrum was measured (Figure EX2.1). The normal ranges of carpal angle in children aged 4–14 years are given in Table EX2.1.

Table EX2.1. Normal range (−2 SD to +2SD) for the carpal angles in children between 4 and 14 years of age. The range for the angle is given separately for white and black children. (After Poznanski et al. 1976)

Age (years)	Range (degrees)	
	White children	Black children
4	110.6–140.4	115.6–143.6
5	111.2–141.4	116.5–145.5
6	111.8–142.4	117.3–147.5
7	112.4–143.4	118.2–149.4
8	113.1–144.3	119.0–151.4
9	113.7–145.3	119.9–153.3
10	114.3–146.3	120.7–155.3
11	114.9–147.3	121.6–157.2
12	115.5–148.3	122.4–159.2
13	116.1–149.3	123.3–161.1
14	116.7–150.3	124.2–163.0

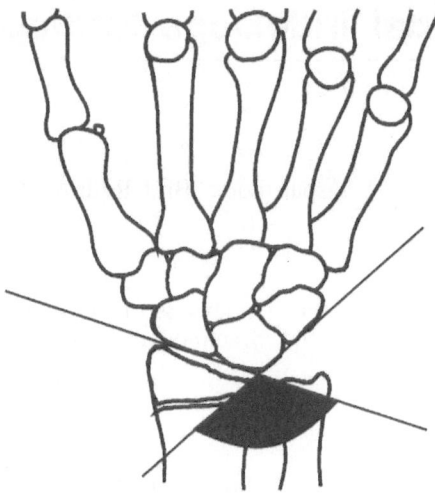

Figure EX2.1. The carpal angle is the angle between the tangent to the proximal edge of the lunate and scaphoid and the tangent to the proximal edge of the lunate and the triquetrum. (After Poznanski et al. 1976.)

EX3 Metacarpal index/age [radiography]

Referenced article:

Walker TM: The normal metacarpal index. Br J Radiol 1979; 52:787.

Background:

The metacarpal index expresses the slenderness of the metacarpals. This is of interest in Marfan's syndrome, but arachnodactyly is also found in other diseases.

Material:

PA radiographs of 2774 children (1470 boys and 1474 girls) who had had their bone age determined at the Bristol Children's Hospital were studied. Films were accepted if there was no evidence of disease affecting the four ulnar metacarpal bones.

Method of measurement:

If all epiphyses in the four ulnar metacarpals were ossified, the axial lengths of the second and third metacarpals were measured from the tip of the metacarpal head, to the apex of the notch at the base. The fourth and fifth metacarpal length was taken as the longest distance from the tip of the head to the most proximal part of the base.

Table EX3.1. Normal range (−2SD to +2SD) for the metacarpal index in normal boys and girls between 1 and 15 years of age. (After Walker 1979)

Age (years)	Boys	Girls
1	4.2–7.0	4.8–7.4
2	4.5–7.3	5.1–7.7
3	4.8–7.5	5.4–8.0
4	5.0–7.7	5.6–8.2
5	5.2–7.9	5.7–8.5
6	5.4–8.1	5.9–8.6
7	5.6–8.2	6.1–8.8
8	5.7–8.4	6.2–9.0
9	5.9–8.5	6.3–9.1
10	6.0–8.6	6.4–9.3
11	6.2–8.7	6.6–9.4
12	6.3–8.9	6.7–9.5
13	6.4–9.0	6.8–9.7
14	6.5–9.1	6.9–9.8
15	6.6–9.2	7.0–9.9

In infants and young children in which all epiphyses were not ossified, the length of each metacarpal was measured as the longest distance from the base to the most distal part of the metaphysis of each bone. In all four metacarpals, the minimal width of the shaft was measured.

The metacarpal index is expressed as the sum of the length of the four ulnar metacarpals, divided by the sum of the width (Table EX3.1).

References:

Joseph MC, Meadow SR: The metacarpal index of infants. Arch Dis Child 1969; 44:515.
Rand TC, Edwards DK, Bay CA, Jones KL: The metacarpal index in normal children. Pediatr Radiol 1980; 9:31.
Walker TM, Ashcroft MT: The metacarpal index in Jamaican children and adults; Br J Radiol 1978; 51:338.

EX4   Metacarpophalangeal length/age [radiography]

Referenced article:

Garn SM, Hertzog KP, Poznanski AK, Nagy JM: Metacarpophalangeal length in the evaluation of skeletal malformation. Radiology 1972; 105:375–381.

Background:

The length of the individual phalanges and metacarpal bones may be influenced by several skeletal dysplasias and endocrine disorders. The individual values may be important for diagnosis in some cases and are therefore presented here. However, the combination of the values – the metacarpophalangeal profile patterns – are of more profound diagnostic importance. For evaluation of such profiles, the reader is referred to Poznanski (1984).

Material:

PA radiographs of the hands of healthy children in the Fels longitudinal studies of growth and development were used. There were 150 children of each sex at age 4 years, 124 at age 9 years, and 30–85 at intermediate ages.

Method of assessment:

The axial lengths of the bones were measured as indicated in Table EX4.1. All measurements represented the total bone length, including the epiphysis, with the exception of the 'hook' at the base of the third metacarpal.

Reference:

Poznanski AK: The hand in radiologic diagnosis. With gamuts and pattern profiles, 2nd edn. WB Saunders, Philadelphia, 1984.

EX4.1. Lengths of metacarpals and phalanges of the hand, according to age. The figures are presented as means and SD for each bone and age between 2 and 16 years and adulthood. The normal range (−2SD to +2SD) is of no interest as these values are used for pattern profile analyses where mean and SD form the bases for calculations rather than the normal range. (From Garn et al. 1972; with permission)

Bone		Age (years)									
		2		3		4		5		6	
		Mean	SD	Mean	SD	Mean	SD	Mean	SD	Mean	SD
Males											
Distal	5	8.8	–	8.4	0.6	9.0	0.7	9.9	0.6	10.7	0.6
	4	9.2	0.7	9.9	0.8	10.5	0.8	11.5	0.9	12.3	0.9
	3	8.7	0.9	9.5	0.8	10.2	0.8	11.1	0.8	11.8	0.9
	2	8.2	0.5	8.8	1.1	9.1	0.8	10.1	0.9	10.8	0.9
	1	11.1	0.6	12.3	0.8	13.2	0.1	14.4	0.9	15.4	0.9
Middle	5	8.8	0.9	9.8	0.8	10.6	1.0	11.2	1.0	12.0	1.0
	4	13.5	0.9	14.5	1.0	15.8	0.9	16.7	0.9	17.7	1.0
	3	14.1	0.8	15.1	1.1	16.5	1.0	17.6	1.0	18.7	1.1
	2	11.2	0.8	12.3	1.1	13.5	1.0	14.4	0.9	15.3	1.0
Proximal	5	16.1	0.7	17.8	0.9	19.2	1.0	20.6	1.0	21.8	1.0
	4	20.5	0.9	22.8	1.0	24.7	1.2	26.4	1.2	27.9	1.3
	3	21.8	1.0	24.2	1.1	26.3	1.4	28.1	1.4	29.8	1.4
	2	19.5	1.0	21.9	1.2	23.7	1.3	25.4	1.4	26.8	1.5
	1	15.2	–	15.9	1.1	17.2	1.1	18.3	1.2	19.6	1.2
Metacarpal	5	23.9	1.0	26.3	1.5	28.9	1.9	32.1	2.2	34.6	2.2
	4	25.5	1.1	28.9	1.5	31.7	2.1	35.0	2.5	37.9	2.7
	3	28.6	1.3	32.3	1.8	35.6	2.3	39.3	2.8	42.6	2.9
	2	30.6	1.5	34.5	1.7	37.9	2.3	41.6	2.7	44.9	2.9
	1	19.6	1.3	22.0	1.2	24.1	1.6	26.7	1.6	29.0	1.7

Table EX4.1. *(continued)*

Bone		Age (years)									
		2		3		4		5		6	
		Mean	SD	Mean	SD	Mean	SD	Mean	SD	Mean	SD
Females											
Distal	5	7.8	0.6	8.4	0.6	9.1	0.7	9.9	0.7	10.6	0.8
	4	9.1	0.7	9.9	0.7	10.6	0.8	11.5	0.9	12.4	1.0
	3	8.8	0.7	9.9	0.8	10.2	0.7	11.1	0.9	12.2	1.3
	2	8.0	0.8	8.6	0.7	9.4	0.7	10.1	0.8	10.9	0.9
	1	11.3	0.8	12.5	0.8	13.2	0.8	14.4	1.0	15.4	1.1
Middle	5	9.0	1.2	9.8	1.1	10.5	1.1	11.1	1.1	12.2	1.2
	4	13.5	0.9	14.9	1.0	15.8	1.1	16.9	1.2	18.1	1.3
	3	14.2	0.9	15.6	1.1	16.6	1.2	17.9	1.2	19.2	1.3
	2	11.6	0.9	12.8	1.0	13.6	1.1	14.8	1.1	16.0	1.2
Proximal	5	16.3	1.0	17.9	1.1	19.1	1.1	20.6	1.3	22.0	1.4
	4	20.7	1.1	22.9	1.3	24.6	1.3	26.3	1.5	28.2	1.7
	3	22.2	1.2	24.5	1.3	26.4	1.4	28.3	1.8	30.4	1.8
	2	20.1	1.2	22.3	1.3	24.0	1.8	25.8	1.7	27.7	1.7
	1	14.9	1.0	16.3	1.1	17.2	1.3	18.8	1.3	20.2	1.3
Metacarpal	5	23.7	1.5	26.9	2.1	29.4	1.8	32.6	2.0	35.1	2.1
	4	26.0	1.9	29.6	2.7	32.2	2.0	35.6	2.5	38.4	2.7
	3	29.4	2.1	33.4	2.9	36.3	2.2	40.3	2.7	43.3	3,1
	2	31.3	1.9	35.2	2.7	38.2	2.3	42.2	2.7	45.6	3.2
	1	19.9	1.6	22.7	1.6	24.8	1.7	27.3	1.8	29.6	1.9

Table EX4.1. *(continued)*

		Age (years)									
		7		8		9		10		11	
Bone		Mean	SD	Mean	SD	Mean	SD	Mean	SD	Mean	SD
Males											
Distal	5	11.4	0.8	12.2	0.9	12.6	1.0	13.5	0.9	14.2	0.9
	4	13.1	1.0	13.9	1.0	14.4	1.0	15.3	1.2	16.1	1.2
	3	12.7	1.0	13.4	1.0	14.0	1.0	14.8	1.2	15.6	1.2
	2	11.6	1.0	12.4	1.0	13.0	1.0	13.7	1.1	14.3	1.1
	1	16.5	1.0	17.4	1.0	17.9	1.2	19.0	1.2	19.7	1.2
Middle	5	12.7	1.1	13.5	1.1	14.3	1.2	15.0	1.2	15.7	1.4
	4	18.7	1.1	19.8	1.1	20.9	1.3	21.6	1.4	22.6	1.5
	3	19.8	1.2	20.9	1.2	22.0	1.4	22.9	1.4	24.0	1.4
	2	16.1	1.1	17.1	1.1	18.1	1.2	18.8	1.2	19.8	1.8
Proximal	5	23.0	1.1	24.2	1.3	25.2	1.5	26.4	1.5	27.6	1.7
	4	29.5	1.4	31.0	1.6	32.3	1.9	33.9	1.8	35.3	2.0
	3	31.5	1.6	33.2	1.8	34.7	2.2	36.1	1.9	37.8	2.3
	2	28.3	1.6	29.7	1.8	31.4	1.9	32.5	1.9	33.9	2.1
	1	20.8	1.3	21.8	1.3	23.1	1.5	24.2	1.4	25.4	1.6
Metacarpal	5	36.7	2.1	38.8	2.5	40.6	2.5	42.7	2.9	44.6	2.8
	4	40.1	2.5	42.2	3.1	44.1	2.8	46.5	3.5	48.4	3.1
	3	45.3	2.8	47.6	3.5	49.8	3.0	52.3	3.7	54.6	3.4
	2	47.7	2.8	50.2	3.4	52.6	3.0	55.0	3.9	57.3	3.5
	1	30.9	1.8	32.7	2.1	34.4	2.1	36.3	2.3	38.2	2.4

Table EX4.1. *(continued)*

		Age (years)								
		7		8		9		10		11	
Bone		Mean	SD	Mean	SD	Mean	SD	Mean	SD	Mean	SD
Females											
Distal	5	11.4	0.9	12.1	1.0	12.7	1.1	13.5	1.2	14.2	1.3
	4	13.2	1.1	14.0	1.1	14.4	1.2	15.5	1.4	16.2	1.4
	3	12.7	1.1	13.5	1.1	14.1	1.1	15.0	1.4	15.8	1.3
	2	11.7	1.0	12.3	1.1	13.1	1.1	13.8	1.4	14.4	1.3
	1	16.3	1.2	17.3	1.3	17.8	1.3	19.0	1.6	20.0	1.7
Middle	5	12.9	1.3	13.6	1.4	14.2	1.4	15.2	1.6	16.2	1.7
	4	19.1	1.4	20.1	1.4	20.9	1.5	22.2	1.7	23.4	1.8
	3	20.3	1.4	21.4	1.4	22.1	1.6	23.6	1.8	24.9	1.9
	2	16.8	1.3	17.8	1.4	18.1	1.5	19.6	1.7	20.6	1.8
Proximal	5	23.1	1.6	24.4	1.6	25.2	1.6	27.1	2.0	28.7	2.1
	4	29.7	1.9	31.2	2.0	32.4	2.0	34.5	2.4	36.5	2.5
	3	32.1	2.0	33.7	2.2	35.0	2.2	37.3	2.6	39.5	2.7
	2	29.2	1.9	30.7	2.0	31.5	2.4	34.0	2.4	35.9	2.6
	1	21.4	1.5	22.7	1.6	23.5	2.0	25.5	2.1	27.2	2.3
Metacarpal	5	37.2	2.4	39.4	2.5	40.8	2.5	43.8	2.8	46.3	2.9
	4	40.5	2.8	43.1	3.0	44.3	2.8	47.5	3.5	50.2	3.8
	3	45.8	3.1	48.7	3.2	49.9	3.2	53.6	3.8	56.5	4.0
	2	48.1	3.3	51.2	3.3	52.6	3.4	56.6	4.1	59.9	4.3
	1	31.5	3.0	33.5	2.1	34.8	2.4	37.4	2.6	39.7	3.0

Table EX4.1. *(continued)*

		Age (years)									
		12		13		14		15		16	
Bone		Mean	SD	Mean	SD	Mean	SD	Mean	SD	Mean	SD
Males											
Distal	5	15.0	0.9	15.8	0.9	16.8	1.0	17.6	1.1	17.9	1.0
	4	17.0	1.3	17.8	1.4	18.8	1.3	19.6	1.4	20.0	1.3
	3	16.4	1.2	17.1	1.3	18.2	1.3	19.0	1.4	19.3	1.4
	2	15.0	1.0	15.7	1.4	16.7	1.2	17.5	1.2	17.8	1.3
	1	20.6	1.3	21.7	1.4	22.8	1.3	24.1	1.4	24.5	1.4
Middle	5	16.5	1.5	17.5	1.5	18.9	1.6	19.9	1.4	20.5	1.4
	4	23.6	1.5	24.8	1.7	26.5	1.6	27.7	1.5	28.4	1.5
	3	24.9	1.4	26.3	1.6	28.0	1.5	29.2	1.5	30.0	1.6
	2	20.4	1.3	21.6	1.6	23.2	1.5	24.3	1.5	25.0	1.5
Proximal	5	28.9	2.0	30.5	2.4	32.9	2.4	34.7	2.0	35.6	1.8
	4	37.0	2.4	38.8	2.8	41.6	2.8	43.7	2.6	44.9	2.3
	3	39.5	2.6	41.5	2.9	44.4	2.8	46.6	2.5	47.8	2.4
	2	35.5	2.4	37.2	2.6	39.8	2.6	41.8	2.2	42.8	2.0
	1	26.7	2.0	28.5	2.2	30.9	2.2	32.9	1.8	33.8	1.5
Metacarpal	5	47.1	3.2	49.1	4.0	52.2	3.9	55.4	3.6	57.1	2.8
	4	51.0	3.7	53.1	4.6	56.4	4.5	59.5	4.1	61.5	3.7
	3	57.3	4.0	59.5	5.1	63.1	4.9	66.7	4.4	68.7	4.1
	2	60.6	3.9	63.3	5.1	67.1	4.8	70.6	4.3	73.2	3.8
	1	40.2	2.7	42.5	3.0	45.1	2.8	47.6	2.6	48.8	2.3

Table EX4.1. (continued)

Bone		12		13		Age (years) 14		15		16	
		Mean	SD	Mean	SD	Mean	SD	Mean	SD	Mean	SD
Females											
Distal	5	15.0	1.3	15.4	1.3	15.6	1.3	15.9	1.4	15.9	1.4
	4	17.1	1.4	17.6	1.2	17.9	1.3	18.0	1.4	18.0	1.3
	3	16.6	1.4	17.1	1.4	17.3	1.3	17.6	1.5	17.5	1.4
	5	15.2	1.5	15.7	1.5	15.8	1.5	16.1	1.6	16.0	1.6
	1	20.9	1.7	21.4	1.6	21.7	1.6	22.0	1.7	22.0	1.7
Middle	5	17.2	1.7	17.9	1.8	18.1	1.6	18.4	1.7	18.5	1.7
	4	24.7	1.8	25.7	1.9	25.9	1.6	26.3	1.8	26.4	1.8
	3	26.2	1.9	27.2	2.0	27.5	1.7	28.1	1.8	28.0	1.9
	2	21.8	1.9	22.7	1.8	23.0	1.8	23.5	1.8	23.3	1.9
Proximal	5	30.5	2.2	31.9	2.2	32.3	2.1	32.9	2.2	32.8	2.3
	4	38.8	2.6	40.3	2.5	40.9	2.3	41.5	2.5	41.6	2.6
	3	41.7	2.8	43.5	2.8	44.1	2.4	44.8	2.6	44.8	2.7
	2	38.0	2.6	39.5	2.6	39.9	2.4	40.6	2.6	40.6	2.6
	1	29.2	2.4	30.6	2.2	31.1	1.9	31.8	2.0	31.7	2.1
Metacarpal	5	48.7	2.9	50.8	2.8	52.1	2.8	52.6	3.0	52.8	3.0
	4	52.8	3.7	55.1	3.6	56.2	3.6	56.9	3.6	57.2	3.9
	3	59.5	4.2	62.1	4.0	63.4	3.9	63.9	3.9	64.3	4.0
	2	63.2	4.4	66.2	4.2	67.4	3.9	68.1	4.2	68.6	4.3
	1	42.0	3.0	43.8	2.7	44.4	2.5	45.3	2.4	45.0	2.8

EX5 Dimensions of distal femoral epiphysis [radiography]

Referenced article:

Schlesinger AE, Poznanski AK, Pudlowski RM, Millar EA: Distal femoral epiphysis: normal standards for thickness and application to bone dysplasias. Radiology 1986; 159:515.

Background:

Flattening of the epiphysis of the long bones is seen in several skeletal dysplasias. In early or subtle cases it may be difficult to assess whether the epiphysis is flattened or not. Normal standards are therefore of value.

Material:

AP radiographs of the knee from 640 normal children from the Fels Research Institute, Yellowsprings, Ohio, were studied. There were 40 boys and 40 girls in each age group (1.5, 3, 5, 7, 9, 11, 13 and 15 years of age).

Method of assessment:

Epiphyseal height, epiphyseal width and metaphyseal width were measured according to Figure EX5.1. Normal ranges for the relationships between epiphyseal height and epiphyseal width and metaphyseal width are given in Tables EX5.1 and EX5.2.

Table EX5.1. Normal range ($-2SD$ to $+2SD$) for distal femoral epiphyseal height (H) (mm) related to the femoral metaphyseal width (FM). The table is valid for children up to 15 years of age and of both sexes. As an example, a normal child with a femoral metaphyseal width of 68 mm has a 96% probability of having an epiphyseal height of 19.3–25.2 mm. (After Schlesinger et al. 1986)

Femoral metaphyseal width (mm)	Femoral epiphyseal height (mm)				
		+1	+2	+3	+4
35	7.7–12.4	8.0–12.7	8.3–13.0	8.6–13.3	9.0–13.7
40	9.3–14.0	9.6–14.3	9.9–14.6	10.3–15.0	10.6–15.3
45	10.9–15.6	11.2–15.9	11.6–16.3	11.9–16.6	12.2–16.9
50	12.6–17.3	12.9–17.6	13.2–17.9	13.5–18.2	13.9–18.8
55	14.4–19.3	14.8–19.8	15.2–20.4	15.6–20.9	16.0–21.5
60	16.4–22.0	16.8–22.5	17.2–23.1	17.7–23.6	18.0–23.9
65	18.3–24.2	18.6–24.6	19.0–24.9	19.3–25.2	19.6–25.5
70	19.9–25.9	20.2–26.2	20.6–26.5	20.9–26.8	21.2–27.1
75	21.5–27.5	21.9–27.8	22.2–28.1	22.5–28.4	22.8–28.8
80	23.1–29.1	23.5–29.4	23.8–29.7	24.1–30.0	24.4–30.4
85	24.8–30.7	25.1–31.0	25.4–31.3	25.7–31.7	26.0–32.0

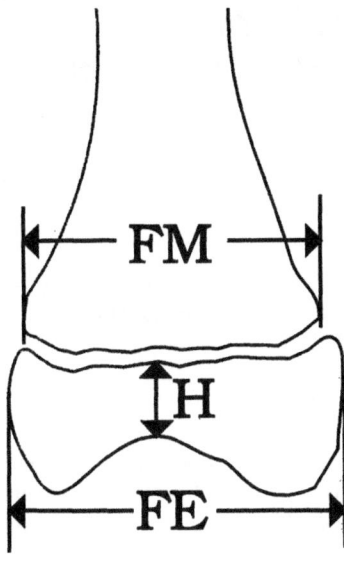

Figure EX5.1. Measurements for evaluation of epiphyseal dimensions. FM, femoral metaphyseal width; FE, femoral epiphyseal width; H, femoral epiphyseal height. (After Schlesinger et al. 1986.)

Table EX5.2. Normal range (−2SD to +2SD) for distal femoral epiphyseal height (H) (mm) related to the femoral epiphyseal width (FE). The table is valid for children up to 15 years of age and for both sexes. As an example a normal child with a femoral epiphyseal width of 68 mm has a 96% probability of having an epiphyseal height of 18.0 to 23.5 mm. (After Schlesinger et al. 1986)

Femoral epiphyseal width (mm)	Femoral epiphyseal height (mm)				
		+1	+2	+3	+4
20	8.9–12.8	9.0–12.9	9.2–13.1	9.4–13.3	9.6–13.5
25	9.8–13.7	10.0–13.9	10.2–14.1	10.4–14.3	10.6–14.5
30	10.8–14.7	10.9–14.8	11.1–15.0	11.3–15.2	11.5–15.4
35	11.7–15.6	11.9–15.8	12.1–16.0	12.3–16.2	12.5–16.4
40	12.7–16.6	12.8–16.7	13.0–16.9	13.2–17.1	13.4–17.3
45	13.6–17.5	13.8–17.7	14.0–17.9	14.2–18.1	14.4–18.3
50	14.6–18.5	14.7–18.6	14.9–18.8	15.0–19.1	15.1–19.4
55	15.2–19.7	15.2–20.0	15.3–20.3	15.4–20.6	15.5–21.0
60	15.7–21.2	16.0–21.5	16.3–21.8	16.6–22.1	16.8–22.3
65	17.1–22.6	17.4–22.9	17.7–23.2	18.0–23.5	18.2–23.7
70	18.5–24.0	18.8–24.3	19.1–24.6	19.3–24.8	19.6–25.1
75	19.9–25.4	20.2–25.7	20.5–26.0	20.7–26.2	21.0–26.5
80	21.3–26.8	21.6–27.1	21.8–27.3	22.1–27.6	22.4–27.9
85	22.7–28.2	23.0–28.5	23.2–28.7	23.5–29.0	23.8–29.3
90	24.1–29.6	24.3–29.8	24.6–30.1	24.9–30.4	25.2–30.7

EX6 Tibiofemoral and metaphyseal–diaphyseal angle/age [radiography]

Referenced article:

Levine AM, Drennan JC: Physiological bowing and tibia vara. The metaphyseal–diaphyseal angle in the measurement of bowleg deformities. J Bone Joint Surg 1982; 61-A:1158.

Background:

Bowleg deformity is common among pediatric orthopaedic patients, covering a wide spectrum from mild physiological bowing to pronounced tibia vara. The present measurements allow early and accurate detection of pathological bowleg deformity.

Material:

AP radiographs of the legs of 52 children with physiological bowing were studied. The examination was performed in the upright weight-bearing position, with AP projection.

Method of assessment:

The tibiofemoral angle and the metaphyseal–diaphyseal angle were determined as shown in Figure EX6.1. Normal ranges are given in Table EX6.1.

Table EX6.1. Normal range ($-2SD$ to $+2SD$) for the tibiofemoral and metaphyseal–diaphyseal angles of the knee in children between 11 and 30 months of age expressed in degrees of varus. (After Levine and Drennan 1982)

Age (months)	Range (degrees)	
	Tibiofemoral angle	Metaphyseal–diaphyseal angle
11–20	6.6 to 34.2	−0.5 to 10.7
21–30	−0.2 to 35.0	−2.5 to 9.9

78

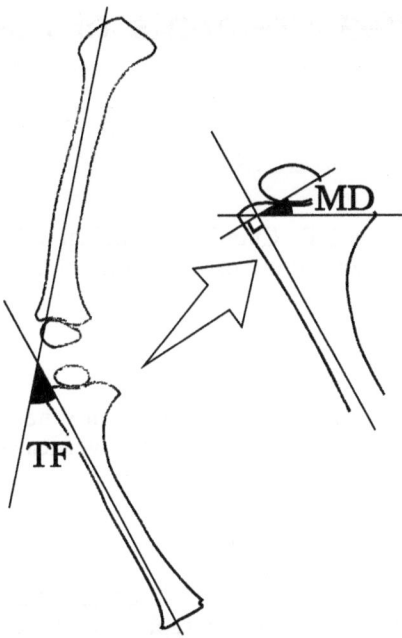

Figure EX6.1. Tibiofemoral and metaphyseal–diaphyseal angles. TF, tibiofemoral angle = the angle between lines drawn along the longitudinal axes of the tibia and femur; MD, metaphyseal–diaphyseal angle = the angle between a line drawn perpendicular to the long axis of the tibia, and another drawn through the two peaks of the metaphysis. (After Levine and Drennan 1982.)

References:

Bateson EM: The relationship between Blount's disease and bowlegs. Br J Radiol 1968; 41:107.
Salenius P, Vankka E: The development of the tibiofemoral angle in children. J Bone Joint Surg 1975; 57-A:529.

EX7 Angle measurements of the foot/age [radiography]

Referenced article:

Van der Wilde R, Staheli LT, Chew DE, Malagon V: Measurements on radiographs of the foot in normal infants and children. J Bone Joint Surg 1988; 70-A:407.

Background:

Normal standards for angular measurements are necessary for adequate evaluation of foot deformities such as club-foot, vertical talus and metatarsus adductus.

Material:

AP and lateral radiographs of the foot of 74 normal infants and children, aged 6–127 months were studied. The radiographs were obtained during weight-bearing. Three projections were obtained: AP, lateral in neutral position, and lateral in maximal dorsiflexion. For the AP projections, the knee was flexed and the central beam was directed towards the head of the talus. For the lateral projections, the central beam was directed towards the talus, and the cassette was held perpendicular to the beam.

Methods of assessment (Figure EX7.1):

On the AP radiographs, three angles were measured: the talocalcaneal angle, the calcaneus/fifth metatarsal angle and the talus/first metatarsal angle.

On the lateral radiograph in neutral position, five angles were measured: the talocalcaneal angle, the tibiocalcaneal angle, the tibiotalar angle, the talus/first metatarsal angle, and the talo-horizontal angle.

In the lateral projection in maximal dorsiflexion, two angles were measured: the talocalcaneal and the tibiocalcaneal angle.

The talocalcaneal index was calculated by adding the values for the anteroposterior and lateral talocalcaneal angles.

Normal ranges for these angle measurements are given in Table EX7.1.

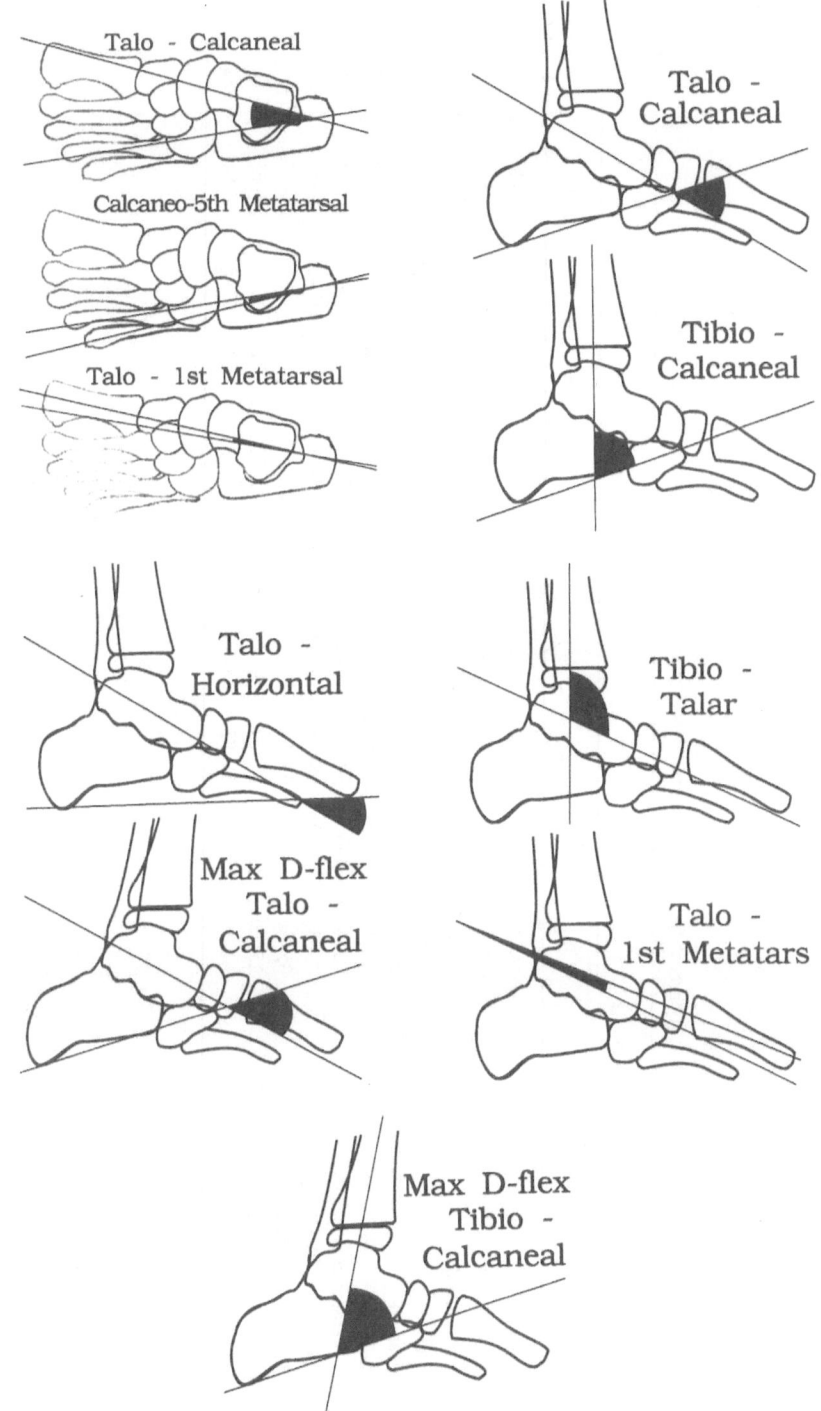

Figure EX7.1. Lines drawn on the AP or lateral radiographs to obtain the angles given in Table EX7.1.

81

Table EX7.1. Normal range (−2SD to +2SD) (degrees) for angle measurements of the foot. (After Van der Wilder et al. 1988)

Type of angle	Age (years)									
	0	1	2	3	4	5	6	7	8	9
AP talocalcaneal	28–57	27–53	27–50	26–47	25–44	23–42	21–40	18–38	15–36	11–34
AP calc./5th metatarsal	−9–14	−10–12	−10–10	−10–9	−10–8	−10–8	−10–9	−9–11	−9–12	−8–15
AP talo/1st metatarsal	9–31	5–28	2–26	−1–25	−3–23	−6–22	−7–21	−8–19	−9–18	−10–17
Lat. talocalcaneal	23–55	27–56	29–57	32–57	33–57	34–56	33–55	32–55	31–54	29–52
Lat. tibiocalcaneal	60–96	58–91	57–87	56–84	56–81	57–78	58–76	60–75	62–74	64–74
Lat. tibiotalar	86–145	90–137	95–131	99–126	101–122	102–120	102–119	100–120	98–122	95–124
Lat. talo/1st metatarsal	−2–40	−3–33	−4–29	−4–25	−5–22	−5–19	−5–18	−6–17	−6–18	−7–18
Lat. talo-horizontal	13–55	16–50	18–46	19–42	20–39	20–37	19–36	17–35	16–35	14–36
Max. dorsiflex. lat. talocalcaneal	35–56	34–55	33–54	33–53	32–53	32–52	31–52	31–51	31–51	30–51
Max. dorsiflex. lat. tibiocalcaneal	25–60	26–65	27–69	29–71	30–73	32–72	34–71	36–69	38–65	40–60
Talocalcaneal index	61–101	65–99	66–97	66–95	65–93	63–91	61–89	57–87	52–84	46–82

EX8 Muscle cylinder ratio in infancy [radiography]

Referenced article:

Litt RE, Altman DH: Significance of the muscle cylinder ratio in infancy. AJR 1967; 100:80.

Background:

Decrease or increase of the muscle mass and subcutaneous fat may appear in a wide spectrum of diseases. Such changes may be expressed as an alteration in the relationship between the muscle mass and subcutaneous fat in the extremities.

Material:

AP radiographs of the lower extremities of 300 normal infants were studied.

Method of assessment:

At midfemur and midthigh, the transverse diameter of the leg (total cylinder diameter, TCD), and the transverse diameter of the muscles (muscle diameter, MD) is measured.

The muscle cylinder ratio (MCR) (Table EX8.1) is calculated according to the formula:

$$MCR = MD/TCD$$

Table EX8.1. Normal value of MCR ($-2SD$ to $+2SD$). (After Litt and Altman 1967)

0.64–0.72

EX9 Limb bone length ratios/age [radiography]

Referenced article:

Robinow M, Chumlea WC: Standards for limb bone length ratios in children. Radiology 1982; 143:433.

Background:

Disproportion between the different large long bones is seen in several skeletal malformations. In many syndromes the disproportion is so obvious that measurements are unnecessary, but the present method may be used to give 'disproportionate profiles' in borderline cases, as well as to express numerically the rhizomelic and mesomelic dwarfism.

Material:

Radiographs of the extremities were obtained at regular intervals in 823 individuals from the age of 2 months to 15 years in the Child Research Council Study, Denver, Colorado, between 1935 and 1967.

Table EX9.1. Normal range (−2SD to +2SD) for limb bone length ratio in children between 0.2 and 15 years of age. The diaphyseal bone length ratio is given for the ages 0–12 years, and the total bone length ratio is given for the age-range 10–15 years. (After Robinow and Chumlea 1982)

Age (years)	Radius Humerus	Tibia Femur	Humerus Femur	Radius Tibia
Diaphyseal bone length ratio				
0.2 < 0.5	0.74–0.90	0.73–0.89	0.73–0.93	0.74–0.94
0.5 < 1.0	0.73–0.85	0.75–0.87	0.73–0.85	0.71–0.83
1.0 < 1.5	0.71–0.83	0.77–0.85	0.73–0.81	0.70–0.78
1.5 < 2.0	0.72–0.80	0.77–0.85	0.72–0.80	0.65–0.77
2.0 < 10	0.71–0.79	0.77–0.85	0.65–0.77	0.59–0.71
10 < 12	0.71–0.79	0.78–0.86	0.65–0.73	0.59–0.67
Total bone length ratio				
10–15	0.71–0.79	0.80–0.88	0.63–0.71	0.55–0.63

Methods of assessment:

Diaphyseal bone length was measured from age 2 months to 12 years, and total bone length (diaphyses + epiphyses) from age 10 to 18 years (Table EX9.1). Up to 12 years of age, the length was measured parallel to the long axis from the most proximal edge to the most distal edge of the diaphysis. From 10 years and up the length was measured from the most proximal edge of the epiphysis at one end of the bone to the most distal edge of the epiphysis at the opposite end, care being taken to keep the ruler parallel to the long axis of the bone. Therefore, for ages 10–12 years there are two sets of measurements.

References:

Anderson MS, Messner MB, Green WT: Distributions of lengths of femur and tibia in children from 1 to 18 years of age. J Bone Joint Surg 1964; 46-A:1197.

Maresh MM, Denning J: The growth of the long bones in 80 infants. Child Dev 1939; 10:91.

EX10 Quadriceps muscle thickness and subcutaneous tissue thickness/age [ultrasound]

Referenced article:

Heckmatt JZ, Pier N, Dubowitz V: Measurement of quadriceps muscle thickness and subcutaneous tissue thickness in normal children by real-time ultrasound imaging. J Clin Ultrasound 1988; 16:171.

Background:

Quantitation of muscle thickness is important in evaluation of muscle atrophy and hypertrophy in neuromuscular disease. Earlier, such measurements were performed using radiography (see subsection EX8), but today reproducible techniques are available with ultrasound that avoid radiation hazards.

Material:

Ultrasound examinations in 276 normal children, aged 0–12 years were studied. Using a real-time scanner with a 3.5 or 5 MHz transducer, cross-sectional examinations of the lateral thigh were obtained at a point halfway between the top of the greater trochanter and the knee joint. Measurements were made with the child seated, the knee extended and the muscle relaxed. To minimise compression of tissue, a generous amount of transmission gel was used and the skin outline in the ultrasound image was observed. Oblique scanning was avoided.

Table EX10.1. Normal ranges (−2SD to +2SD) for ultrasonically determined quadriceps muscle and subcutaneous tissue thickness in children from 0 to 12 years of age for each year. Subcutaneous tissue thickness is given separately for boys and girls. (After Heckmatt et al. 1988)

Age (years)	Muscle thickness Both sexes (mm)	Soft tissue thickness (mm)	
		Boys	Girls
0	10.3–18.6	3.1–13.1	3.1–12.2
1	13.3–25.2	3.1–13.4	3.3–12.9
2	14.5–28.0	3.2–13.7	3.5–13.6
3	15.4–30.1	3.3–14.0	3.7–14.4
4	16.2–31.8	3.4–14.4	3.9–15.2
5	16.9–33.4	3.4–14.7	4.1–16.1
6	17.5–34.8	3.5–15.0	4.3–17.0
7	18.1–36.1	3.6–15.4	4.6–18.0
8	18.6–37.3	3.7–15.7	4.8–19.0
9	19.1–38.4	3.8–16.1	5.1–20.1
10	19.6–39.5	3.8–16.5	5.4–21.2
11	20.0–40.5	3.9–16.8	5.7–22.4
12	20.5–41.5	4.0–17.2	6.0–23.7

Method of assessment:

Measurements of the skin to fascia and skin to bone distance were made from the image at the time of scanning, using electronic calipers.

Normal ranges for boys and girls are given in Table EX10.1.

SECTION 5
Bone Mineral Contents

BM1 Cortical metacarpal thickness/age [radiography]

Referenced article:

Garn SM, Poznanski AK, Nagy JM: Bone measurement in the differential diagnosis of osteopenia and osteoporosis. Radiology 1971; 100:509.

Background:

Changes in bone mineral content are reflected in the cortical thickness of the long bones. This measurement is relatively insensitive – small and moderate bone mineral changes are not detected, but the measurements serve as a rough method for evaluation of bone formation and bone loss.

Material:

PA radiographs of the hand of about 700 healthy children of both sexes were studied.

Method of assessment:

Caliper measurements were performed of the total subperiosteal diameter T and the medullary cavity width M of the second metacarpal at its midshaft. The cortical width was expressed as T − M, and the cortical areas as

$$\frac{\pi}{4}(T^2 - M^2)$$

Normal ranges for metacarpal width, cortical thickness and cortical area in boys and girls are given in Tables BM1.1 and BM1.2.

Table BM1.1. Normal range (−2SD to +2SD) for metacarpal width, cortical thickness and cortical area in boys between 1 and 16 years of age. (After Garn et al. 1971)

Age (years)	Metacarpal width (mm)	Cortical width (mm)	Cortical area (mm²)
1	3.8–5.2	0.9–2.1	5.3–11.9
2	4.2–6.0	1.1–2.6	7.4–16.8
3	4.4–6.3	1.4–2.9	9.5–19.3
4	4.6–6.5	1.7–3.2	11.6–21.7
5	4.8–6.8	1.9–3.5	12.9–25.0
6	5.0–7.1	2.1–3.9	14.2–28.3
7	5.2–7.4	2.3–4.1	16.3–31.1
8	5.5–7.7	2.5–4.3	18.3–33.9
9	5.7–8.0	2.7–4.6	20.1–37.8
10	6.0–8.3	2.9–4.9	21.9–41.8
11	6.2–8.7	3.0–5.2	23.4–46.1
12	6.4–9.0	3.1–5.5	24.9–50.4
13	6.7–9.5	3.3–5.9	27.4–57.1
14	7.0–10.1	3.5–6.3	29.8–63.9
15	7.3–10.3	3.9–6.3	34.3–66.4
16	7.7–10.6	4.3–6.3	38.8–68.9

Table BM1.2. Normal range (−2SD to +2SD) for metacarpal width, cortical thickness and cortical area in girls between 1 and 16 years of age. (After Garn et al. 1971)

Age (years)	Metacarpal width (mm)	Cortical width (mm)	Cortical area (mm²)
1	3.6–5.1	0.9–2.1	4.5–12.3
2	4.0–5.9	1.1–2.5	6.5–16.1
3	4.2–6.1	1.3–2.8	8.1–18.5
4	4.4–6.4	1.6–3.0	9.8–21.0
5	4.5–6.6	1.8–3.3	10.0–23.4
6	4.7–6.8	1.9–3.6	12.2–25.8
7	4.9–7.1	2.1–3.8	13.8–28.7
8	5.1–7.4	2.4–4.0	15.5–31.5
9	5.3–7.7	2.5–4.3	16.8–34.7
10	5.5–8.1	2.6–4.5	18.1–37.9
11	5.8–8.4	2.8–4.9	20.3–42.4
12	6.0–8.8	3.0–5.3	22.5–46.9
13	6.3–8.9	3.6–5.6	25.4–50.0
14	6.5–9.0	3.7–6.0	28.2–53.0
15	6.6–9.0	3.8–6.1	28.9–53.6
16	6.6–9.0	3.9–6.3	29.6–54.2

BM2 Cortical mass in neonates [radiography]

Referenced article:

Poznanski AK, Kuhns LR, Guire KE: New standards of cortical mass in the humerus of neonates: a means of evaluating bone loss in the premature infant. Radiology 1980; 134:639.

Background:

There may be considerable bone loss in premature children. The present method, based on measurements of the humeral diaphysis, is practical because it can be applied on standard radiographs of the chest.

Material:

Routine AP chest radiographs of 132 neonates ranging in weight from 500 to 3686 g were included. Their birth weight was appropriate for gestational age. Depending on the position of the arm, the humerus had been exposed either in the AP or the lateral projection.

Method of assessment:

The measurements were obtained above the point where the nutrient foramen enters the humerus. In the AP view the nutrient foramen is clearly seen, and

Table BM2.1. Normal ranges (−2SD and + 2SD) for different cortical measurements of the preterm and neonatal humerus. All values are given for each gestational week from 26 to 40. (After Poznanski et al. 1980)

Gestational age (weeks)	Outside diameter (mm)	Cortical thickness (mm)	Cortical area (mm²)
26	2.6–4.2	1.7–3.1	2.8–13.3
27	2.7–4.3	1.8–3.3	3.8–14.3
28	2.9–4.5	2.0–3.4	4.7–15.3
29	3.0–4.6	2.1–3.5	5.7–16.2
30	3.2–4.8	2.2–3.6	6.6–17.2
31	3.3–4.9	2.3–3.7	7.6–18.1
32	3.5–5.1	2.5–3.9	8.6–19.1
33	3.6–5.3	2.6–4.0	9.5–20.1
34	3.8–5.4	2.7–4.1	10.5–21.0
35	3.9–5.6	2.8–4.2	11.5–22.0
36	4.1–5.7	2.9–4.4	12.4–22.9
37	4.2–5.9	3.1–4.5	13.4–23.9
38	4.4–6.0	3.2–4.6	14.3–24.9
39	4.5–6.2	3.3–4.7	15.3–25.8
40	4.7–6.3	3.4–4.8	16.3–26.8

the measurement was performed just superior to this. In the lateral view the more distal portion of the nutrient canal is seen as a small circle in the centre of the bone. The measurement was taken 2 mm superior to this.

Two measurements were obtained with a direct reading caliper: the outside diameter T and the inner diameter M. From these measurements, the cortical thickness (C) was determined (C = T − M). The cortical area (CA) was calculated as $\pi/4$ $(T^2 - M^2)$.

Normal ranges for the different cortical measurements related to gestational age and birth weight are given in Tables BM2.1 and BM2.2, respectively.

Table BM2.2. Normal ranges (−2SD and +2SD) for different cortical measurements of the preterm and neonatal humerus. All values are given in relation to birth weight between 0.6 and 3.8 kg. (After Poznanski et al. 1980)

Birth weight (kg)	Outside diameter (mm)	Cortical thickness (mm)	Cortical area (mm^2)
0.6	2.6–4.0	1.7–3.1	2.7–12.2
0.7	2.7–4.1	1.8–3.1	3.3–12.8
0.8	2.7–4.2	1.9–3.2	3.8–13.3
0.9	2.8–4.3	1.9–3.2	4.3–13.9
1.0	2.9–4.4	2.0–3.3	4.9–14.4
1.1	3.0–4.5	2.1–3.4	5.4–14.9
1.2	3.1–4.5	2.1–3.4	6.0–15.5
1.3	3.2–4.6	2.2–3.5	6.5–16.0
1.4	3.3–4.7	2.3–3.6	7.0–16.5
1.5	3.3–4.8	2.3–3.6	7.6–17.1
1.6	3.4–4.9	2.4–3.7	8.1–17.6
1.7	3.5–5.0	2.4–3.7	8.6–18.2
1.8	3.6–5.0	2.5–3.8	9.2–18.7
1.9	3.7–5.1	2.6–3.9	9.7–19.2
2.0	3.8–5.2	2.6–3.9	10.2–19.8
2.1	3.8–5.3	2.7–4.0	10.8–20.3
2.2	3.9–5.4	2.8–4.1	11.3–20.8
2.3	4.0–5.5	2.8–4.1	11.9–21.4
2.4	4.1–5.5	2.9–4.2	12.4–21.9
2.5	4.2–5.6	2.9–4.2	12.9–22.4
2.6	4.3–5.7	3.0–4.3	13.5–23.0
2.7	4.3–5.8	3.1–4.4	14.0–23.5
2.8	4.4–5.9	3.1–4.4	14.5–24.1
2.9	4.5–6.0	3.2–4.5	15.1–24.6
3.0	4.6–6.1	3.3–4.6	15.6–25.1
3.1	4.7–6.1	3.3–4.6	16.1–25.7
3.2	4.8–6.2	3.4–4.7	16.7–26.2
3.3	4.8–6.3	3.4–4.7	17.2–26.7
3.4	4.9–6.4	3.5–4.8	17.8–27.3
3.5	5.0–6.5	3.6–4.9	18.3–27.8
3.6	5.1–6.6	3.6–4.9	18.8–28.3
3.7	5.2–6.6	3.7–5.0	19.4–28.9
3.8	5.3–6.7	3.8–5.1	19.9–29.4

BM3 Quantitative spinal mineral analysis [CT]

Referenced article:

Gilsanz V, Verterasian M, Senac MO, Cann CE: Quantitative spinal mineral analysis in children. Ann Radiol 1986; 29:380.

Background:

Radiographic analysis of cortical thickness has been used as a means for evaluation of bone mineral content (see subsections BM1 and BM2). However, this method is relatively insensitive. Today, CT techniques are available that can measure bone mineral content in the spine more accurately.

Material:

CT examinations of the spine in 40 normal children (27 boys and 13 girls), aged 4 months–18 years, were studied. CT examination was occasioned because of a motor vehicle accident.

Method of assessment:

Quantitative CT was performed using a mineral reference standard for simultaneous calibration. Two continuous slices in the midportions of the vertebral bodies L1–L2 were taken at 80 kV, 80 mA. Approximately 4 cm^3 of purely trabecular bone at the midplane of the vertebral bodies was quantified and the results expressed in mineral equivalents of dipotassium hydrogen phosphate in mg/cm^3 (Table BM3.1).

Table BM3.1. Normal range ($-2SD$ to $+2SD$) for the bone mineral content of L1 and L2 in boys and girls between 0.3 and 18 years of age. (After Gilsanz et al. 1986)

	Bone mineral content (mg/cm^3)
Boys	140.4–222.8
Girls	123.7–231.6
All	135.2–225.5

BM4 Bone mineral content at birth [single photon absorptiometry]

Referenced article:

Vyhmeister NR, Linkhart TA: Measurement of humerus and radius bone mineral content in the term and preterm infant. J Pediatr 1988; 113:188.

Background:

Single photon absorptiometry is an established tool for evaluation of bone mineral content. In the adult, the measurement is often performed at the radius. In infants, and especially in very low birth weight infants, measurements performed at the midhumerus may be preferable.

Material:

A total of 148 normal children (term and preterm) were examined within the first week of life.

Method of assessment:

The measurements were made with a digital bone densitometer, with a sealed 200 mCi ^{125}I gamma ray source, and 3.2 mm collimator. All measurements were done with the infant lying supine on the deck of the densitometer. Care was taken to minimise stress to the infant, and normal body temperature was maintained with heating lamps and blankets. All measurements were done in the single scan mode. The measurements on the humerus were performed at the midhumerus site.

Normal ranges for bone mineral content in relation to gestational age and body weight are given in Tables BM4.1 and BM4.2 respectively.

Table BM4.1. Normal range (−2SD to +2SD) for bone mineral content of the humerus in newborn preterm and term infants in relation to gestational age between 25 and 42 weeks. (After Vyhmeister and Linkhart 1988)

Gestational age (weeks)	Bone mineral content (mg/cm³)	Gestational age (weeks)	Bone mineral content (mg/cm³)
25	49–87	35	97–209
26	49–99	36	107–221
27	51–111	37	118–234
28	53–123	38	130–246
29	57–136	39	143–258
30	61–148	40	157–270
31	66–126	41	172–283
32	72–172	42	188–295
33	80–185		
34	88–197		

Table BM4.2. Normal range (−2SD to +2SD) for bone mineral content (mg cm³) of the humerus in newborn preterm and term infants in relation to body weight between 500 and 4400 g. (After Vyhmeister and Linkhart 1988)

Body weight	+0	+100	+200	+300	+400
500	46– 89	47– 95	48–101	49–108	51–114
1000	53–120	55–127	57–133	60–139	62–145
1500	65–152	68–158	71–164	75–170	78–177
2000	82–183	86–189	90–196	94–202	99–208
2500	104–214	109–221	114–227	119–233	125–239
3000	130–246	136–252	142–258	149–264	155–271
3500	162–277	169–283	176–290	183–296	191–302
4000	198–308	206–315	214–321	222–327	231–333

BM5 Bone mineral content/age [single photon absorptiometry]

Referenced article:

Klemm T, Banzer DH, Schneider U: Bone mineral content of the growing skeleton. AJR 1976; 126:1283.

Background:

See subsection BM4.

Material:

A total of 124 normal children (66 boys and 58 girls, aged 3–16 years) were examined for bone mineral content (BMC) of the calcaneus, using single photon absorptiometry.

Method of measurement:

The BMC was expressed in g/cm length unit, and in mg/cm^3 bone volume, indicating the bone density (Table BM5.1).

Table BM5.1. Normal ranges (−2SD to +2SD) for bone mineral density (BMD) and bone mineral content (BMC) in the calcaneus in children between 3 and 15 years old. (After Klemm et al. 1976)

Age (years)	Boys		Girls	
	BMD (mg/cm^3)	BMC (g/cm)	BMD (mg/cm^3)	BMC (g/cm)
3	100–205	0.29–1.10	100–225	0.32–1.22
4	106–212	0.43–1.31	105–231	0.44–1.41
5	112–219	0.56–1.52	111–237	0.55–1.59
6	118–226	0.70–1.74	116–243	0.67–1.77
7	124–232	0.84–1.95	121–249	0.78–1.96
8	130–239	0.97–2.17	126–254	0.90–2.14
9	136–246	1.11–2.38	132–260	1.01–2.32
10	142–253	1.24–2.59	137–266	1.13–2.51
11	148–260	1.38–2.81	142–272	1.25–2.69
12	154–266	1.51–3.02	148–278	1.36–2.88
13	160–273	1.65–3.23	153–284	1.48–3.06
14	165–280	1.79–3.45	158–290	1.59–3.24
15	171–287	1.92–3.66	164–296	1.71–3.43

SECTION 6
The Respiratory Tract

RT1   Adenoidal size/age [radiography]

Referenced article:

Fujioka M, Young LW, Girdany BR: Radiographic evaluation of adenoidal size in children: adenoidal–nasopharyngeal ratio. AJR 1979; 133:401.

Background:

Radiographic evaluation of the nasopharynx is essential for decision of adenoidectomy or tonsillectomy. Several methods for such evaluation have been proposed. The present method is easy to adapt and reliably describes not only the size of the adenoid, but also the patency of the nasopharyngeal airway.

Material:

Lateral radiographs of the nasopharynx, were obtained from 1398 healthy children (872 boys and 596 girls). The focus–film distance was 180 cm.

Method of assessment:

The adenoid measure (A) and the nasopharyngeal measure (N) were obtained as shown in Figure RT1.1. The A/N ratio was calculated (Table RT1.1).

Table RT1.1. Normal range ($-2SD$ to $+2SD$) for the adenoidal–nasopharyngeal ratio in children up to the age of 16 years. (After Fujioka et al. 1979)

Age (years)	Ratio	Age (years)	Ratio
0.1	0.10–0.56	7.5	0.34–0.81
0.4	0.21–0.71	8.5	0.32–0.81
0.8	0.29–0.73	9.5	0.29–0.81
1.3	0.34–0.74	10.5	0.26–0.81
1.8	0.35–0.75	11.5	0.23–0.81
2.5	0.36–0.77	12.5	0.21–0.80
3.5	0.36–0.78	13.5	0.17–0.76
4.5	0.36–0.79	14.5	0.13–0.72
5.5	0.36–0.80	15.5	0.09–0.69
6.5	0.35–0.80		

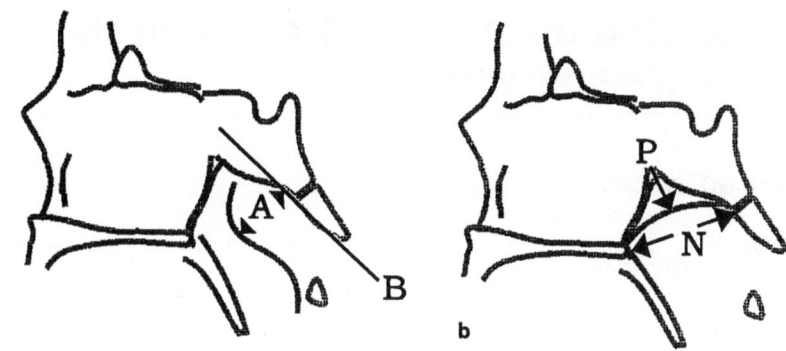

Figure RT1.1. a Adenoidal measurements: B, a line drawn along the straight part of the anterior margin of the basiocciput; A, the perpendicular distance between B and the point of maximal convexity of the adenoid. **b** Nasopharyngeal measurements: N, the distance between the posterior superior edge of the hard palate and the anteroinferior edge the sphenobasioccipital synchondiosis. When this latter point is not clearly seen, it may be determined as the site of crossing between the posteroinferior margin of the lateral pterygoid plates (P) and floor of bony nasopharynx. (After Fujioka et al. 1979.)

RT2 Sagittal diameter of trachea in the newborn [radiography]

Referenced article:

Donaldson SW, Tompsett AC: Tracheal diameter in the normal newborn infant. AJR 1952; 67:785.

Background:

Measurements of the trachea are useful for detection of tracheal abnormalities and in problems with endotracheal intubation, endoscopy and tracheostomy. Tracheal dimensions undergo considerable changes parallel with changes in intraluminal pressure and respiratory phase, as well as body position. The data presented are therefore only valid for the given examination circumstances (see below).

Material:

Lateral radiographs of the neck in 315 normal newborns were studied. Every effort was made to include only those examinations in which the exposure was made at the height of inspiration. Film–focus distance was 36 inches (91.4 cm), and magnification was not corrected for.

Method of assessment:

The sagittal diameter, perpendicular to the tracheal long axis, was measured at the midlevel of the vertebral bodies C5, T1 and T3. Normal ranges are given in Table RT2.1.

Table RT2.1. Normal range (−2SD to +2SD) for the anteroposterior tracheal diameter in the newborn at the level of three selected vertebral body levels. (After Donaldson and Tompsett 1952)

Vertebral level	Tracheal diameter (mm)
C5	3.3–5.9
T1	3.0–4.9
T3	2.4–4.8

RT3   Transverse tracheal diameter/age [radiography]

Referenced article:

Menu Y, Lallemand D: Détermination du diamètre transversal normal de la trachée ches l'enfant. Ann Radiol (Paris) 1981; 24:73.

Background:

See subsection RT2.

Material:

Normal chest films in 170 children aged 1 month–16 years were studied. The film–focus distance was 50 cm. For ages 0–7 years, except in infants, the AP view was used, in the standing position. Above 7 years, the PA view was used. The transverse diameter was measured at two levels: halfway between the glottis and the manubrium sterni, and halfway between the manubrium sterni and the tracheal bifurcation. There was no statistical difference between the two measurements. Normal ranges are given in Table RT3.1.

Table RT3.1. Normal range (−2SD to +2SD) of transverse cervical or thoracic tracheal diameters related to age between 0 and 17 years of age for both sexes. (After Menu and Lallemand 1981)

Age (years)	Diameter (mm)	Age (years)	Diameter (mm)	Age (years)	Diameter (mm)
0	3.5–8.2	1	3.9–8.8	2	4.3–9.4
3	4.7–9.9	4	5.1–10.5	5	5.5–11.1
6	5.9–11.6	7	6.3–12.2	8	6.7–12.8
9	7.1–13.3	10	7.5–13.9	11	7.9–14.5
12	8.3–15.0	13	8.7–15.6	14	9.1–16.2
15	9.5–16.7	16	9.9–17.3	17	10.3–17.9

RT4 Tracheal dimensions/age [CT]

Referenced article:

Griscom TN, Wohl MEB: Dimensions of the growing trachea related to age and gender. AJR 1986; 146:233.

Background:

See subsection RT2.

Material:

CT examinations of 130 children and adolescents who were examined for possible pulmonary metastases were studied. Patients with nearby tumours and local processes likely to affect the trachea were excluded. The patients were examined supine, at relatively low lung volume up to the age of 6 years, and holding their breath near total lung capacity above the age of 6 years. Contiguous, 10 mm CT sections were obtained.

Method of assessment:

Tracheal length as measured from vocal cords to carina was determined from the digital radiograph. Diameters and cross-sectional areas were determined from each section and averaged. Intratracheal volume was calculated by multiplying length by mean cross-sectional area. The length of the trachea, the

Table RT4.1. Normal ranges (−2SD to +2SD) for tracheal measurements in children between 0 and 15 years of age. Both sexes are included. (After Griscom and Wohl 1986)

Age (years)	Length (mm)	AP diameter (mm)	Transverse diameter (mm)	Cross-sectional area (mm^2)
0	39.4– 60.5	3.6– 6.6	4.2– 7.8	3.5– 23.7
1	43.0– 65.8	4.1– 7.2	4.8– 8.3	10.5– 35.3
2	46.6– 71.1	4.7– 7.9	5.3– 8.9	17.4– 46.8
3	50.2– 76.4	5.2– 8.5	5.8– 9.5	24.4– 58.4
4	53.8– 81.8	5.8– 9.2	6.4–10.0	31.3– 70.0
5	57.4– 87.1	6.3– 9.8	6.9–10.6	38.2– 81.5
6	61.0– 92.4	6.9–10.5	7.5–11.1	45.2– 93.1
7	64.6– 97.7	7.4–11.1	8.0–11.7	52.1–104.7
8	68.2–103.0	8.0–11.8	8.5–12.2	59.1–116.2
9	71.8–108.3	8.5–12.4	9.1–12.8	66.0–127.8
10	75.4–113.7	9.1–13.1	9.6–13.3	73.0–139.4
11	78.9–119.0	9.6–13.7	10.1–13.9	79.9–151.0
12	82.5–124.3	10.2–14.4	10.7–14.4	86.9–162.5
13	86.1–129.6	10.8–15.0	11.2–15.0	93.8–174.1
14	89.7–134.9	11.3–15.7	11.8–15.5	100.7–185.7
15	93.3–140.2	11.9–16.3	12.3–16.1	107.7–197.2

mean AP diameter, the mean transverse diameter and the mean cross-sectional area were calculated, according to age (Table RT4.1).

References:

Effmann EL, Fram EK, Vock P, Kirks DR: Tracheal cross-sectional area in children: CT determination. Radiology 1983; 149:137.
Griscom NT: Computed tomographic determination of tracheal dimensions in children and adolescents. Radiology 1982; 145:361.

RT5   Thymus dimensions/age [CT]

Referenced article:

Amour TES, Siegel MJ, Glazer HS, Nadel SN: CT appearances of the normal and abnormal thymus in childhood. J Comput Assist Tomogr 1987; 11:645.

Background:

At CT examination, most abnormal thymuses are obvious at qualitative assessment. However, exact measurements of the thymus may be useful in the diagnosis of infiltrating diseases. The measurements presented here are simple to perform and commonly used (Salonen 1984; Francis 1985).

Material:

CT examinations of 71 chyildren aged 0–19 years were examined. The children had no thymic abnormality, and the examinations were performed for evaluation of the extent of extrathoracic tumours without thymic involvement. The CT scans were obtained in full inspiration in children above 5 years of age, and at resting volume in younger children, using 1 cm intervals with 8 mm collimation.

Method of assessment:

On a transverse scan where each diameter appeared largest, the anteroposterior diameter (AP), the transverse dimension, the width (W) and the thickness (T) were measured according to the Figure RT5.1. Normal ranges are given in Table RT5.1.

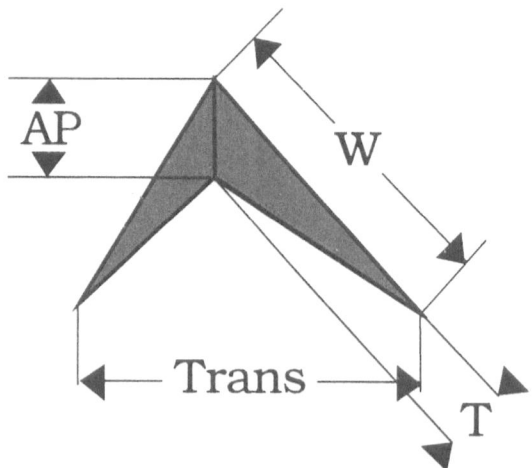

Figure RT5.1. Measurements obtained of thymus gland: AP, anteroposterior dimension; Trans, transverse dimension; W, width (for each lobe); T, thickness (for each lobe). (After Amour et al. 1987.)

Table RT5.1. Normal range (−2SD to +2SD) for some dimensions of the thymus, as well as its right and left lobe. Diameters are given for different age groups for boys and girls together. (After Amour et al. 1987)

Age (years)	AP dimension (cm)	Transverse dimension (cm)	Right lobe		Left lobe	
			Width (cm)	Thickness (cm)	Width (cm)	Thickness (cm)
0–5	0.6–2.6	3.3–5.7	1.3–4.1	0.3–1.5	1.8–5.4	0.4–2.4
6–10	0.3–2.7	2.2–6.2	1.1–3.9	0.0–2.0	1.5–6.3	0.2–1.8
11–15	0.4–3.6	3.4–5.4	1.3–4.1	0.2–1.4	3.1–5.9	0.0–2.0
16–19	0.7–3.1	2.3–5.5	1.1–3.9	0.3–1.1	2.4–6.0	0.0–1.6

References:

Francis IR, Glazer GM, Bookstein FL, Gross BH: The thymus: reexamination of age-related changes in size and shape. AJR 1985; 145:249–254.

Salonen OLM, Kivisaari ML, Somar KJ: Computed tomography of the thymus of children under 10 years. Pediatr Radiol 1984; 14:373–375.

RT6 The width of the paratracheal stripe [radiography]

Referenced article:

Savoca CJ, Brasch RC. Gooding CA, Gamsu G: The right paratracheal stripe in children. Pediatr Radiol 1978; 6:203.

Background:

The right paratracheal stripe is defined as the thin stripe of water density seen on frontal chest radiographs between the air in the trachea and the adjacent right lung. The paratracheal stripe comprises tracheal, mediastinal and pleural tissue, and a widening of the stripe indicates disease in any of these structures. It should be noted that it is not possible to identify the paratracheal stripe in a considerable percentage of cases (Neufang and Benz-Bohm 1989).

Material:

PA radiographs from 100 patients, 5–15 years old were studied. None of the children had chest-related disease and all radiographs were normal.

Method of assessment:

The right paratracheal stripe was measured at a level 2 cm above the superior extent of the azygos arch, or, if the azygos arch was not visible, 2 cm above the superior margin of the right main bronchus at its origin. The normal range is given in Table RT6.1.

Table RT6.1. Normal range ($-2SD$ to $+2SD$) for the right paratracheal stripe thickness in children of both sexes between 5 months and 15 years of age. (After Savoca et al. 1978)

Normal range	0.8–3.2 mm

Reference:

Neufang KFR, Benz-Bohm G: Pleuromediastinale Linien beim Säugling, Kind und Jugendlichen – ein Beitrag zur Kenntnis der normalen Röntgenanatomie der Mediastinalgrenzen. Fortschr Röntgenstr 1989; 151:257–262.

SECTION 7
The Cardiovascular System

CV1 Cardiac volume according to body surface area [radiography]

Referenced article:

Ghaffarpour R, Ringertz H, Rudhe U, Wallgren G: Röntgenologisk hjärtvolymbestämning hos barn. (Radiographic measurement of cardiac volume in children). Läkartidningen 1966; 63:3764 (Swedish Medical Journal).

Background:

When evaluated by an experienced pediatric radiologist, a rough estimation of the cardiac size may be appropriate for clinical use. However, for the more inexperienced radiologist, and for scientific use, three-dimensional measurements provide the most accurate results. In the present method, the cardiac volume is related to the total body surface area. The relative volume in cm^3/m^2 body surface area should be avoided in children, as it implies large variation during growth (Dahlström and Ringertz 1984).

Material:

Chest radiographs in 393 children, aged newborn–15 years were studied. In retrospect, all children were regarded clinically as normal, and the chest radiographs were normal. Children below the age of 5–6 years were examined supine (AP) and in the left lateral decubitus, whereas children above 6 years of age were examined standing, PA and lateral. The focus–film distance for the supine examinations was 105 cm, and for the standing examinations 175 cm.

Method of assessment:

On the AP or PA films, the cardiac silhouette is drawn as close to an ellipse as possible, and the long (A) and short (B) axes of this ellipse measured. On the lateral film, the greatest horizontal depth of the heart (C) is measured Figure CV1.1.

The cardiac volume is calculated according to the ellipsoid formula:

$$\text{Volume (V)} = F \times A \times B \times C$$

Factor F includes correction both for the ellipsoid formula constant and the magnification factor. Factor F varies with the focus–film distance and the mean distance between the heart and the chest wall. Factor F is found in Tables CV1.1 and CV1.2.

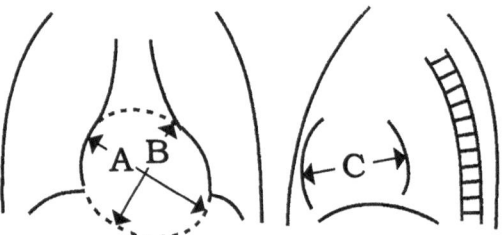

Figure CV1.1. The measurements performed to obtain the length of the three axes of the heart.

Table CV1.1. Mean distance heart–outer chest wall according to age. To be used in Table CV1.2. (After Ghaffarpour et al. 1966)

	AP	PA
Newborn	6 cm	(4 cm)
Supine (0–4–6 years)	10 cm	(6 cm)
Standing (4–11 years)	12 cm	8 cm
Standing (11–15 years)	(14 cm)	10 cm

Table CV1.2. Factor F (including the ellipsoid formula constant and the magnification factor) according to focus–film distance and heart–film distance. (After Ghaffarpour et al. 1966)

Heart–film distance (distance heart–outer chest wall (Table CV1.1) + distance outer chest wall–film (cm)	Focus–film distance (cm)				
	100	125	150	175	200
6	0.43	0.45	0.46	0.47	0.48
8	0.41	0.43	0.44	0.46	0.46
10	0.38	0.41	0.43	0.44	0.45
12	0.36	0.39	0.41	0.42	0.43
14	0.33	0.37	0.39	0.41	0.42
16	0.31	0.35	0.37	0.39	0.41
18	0.29	0.33	0.36	0.38	0.39
20	0.27	0.31	0.34	0.36	0.38
22	0.25	0.29	0.33	0.35	0.37

Table CV1.3. Normal range of cardiac volume ($-2SD$ to $+2SD$) (ml) calculated according to the formula $V = F \times A \times B \times C$, for children of both sexes in the decubitus position during the examination. The volume is related to body surface area according to Du Bois and Du Bois (1916) (Appendix 1). Example: a normal child 72 cm tall of 10 kg has a body surface area of 0.42 m^2 and a 96% probability of having a cardiac volume between 91 and 187 ml. (After Ghaffarpour et al. 1966)

Body surface area (m^2)	—	+ 0.01	+ 0.02	+ 0.03	+ 0.04
0.10	0–54	0–59	0–63	0–68	0–72
0.15	0–77	0–81	0–85	0–90	2–94
0.20	6–98	10–102	14–107	18–111	22–115
0.25	26–119	30–123	34–128	38–132	42–136
0.30	46–140	49–144	53–148	57–152	61–156
0.35	65–160	69–164	72–168	76–172	80–176
0.40	83–179	87–183	91–187	94–191	98–195
0.45	102–198	105–202	109–206	112–210	116–213
0.50	119–217	123–221	126–224	130–228	133–231
0.55	137–235	140–238	143–242	147–245	150–249
0.60	153–252	157–256	160–259	163–262	167–266
0.65	170–269	173–272	176–276	179–279	183–282
0.70	186–286	189–289	192–292	195–295	198–298
0.75	201–301	204–304	207–308	210–311	213–314

The total body surface area according to weight and length is given in Appendix 1 (Du Bois and Du Bois 1916). The cardiac volume calculated according to the formula $V = F \times A \times B \times C$, and related to the total body surface area is given in Tables CV1.3–CV1.5.

Practical use:

1. Perform measurements A, B and C on the chest films.
2. Estimate distance heart–outer chest wall (Table CV1.1).
3. Estimate factor F (Table CV1.2).
4. Calculate cardiac volume ($F \times A \times B \times C$).
5. Estimate body surface area (Appendix 1).
6. Relate cardiac volume to body surface area (Tables CV1.3–CV1.5).

Table CV1.4. Normal range ($-2SD$ to $+2SD$) for cardiac volume (ml) calculated according to the formula $V = F \times A \times B \times C$, for girls standing during the examination. The volume is related to body surface area according to Du Bois and Du Bois (1916) (Appendix 1). (After Ghaffarpour et al. 1966)

Body surface area (m²)	—	+ 0.05	+ 0.10	+ 0.15	+ 0.20
0.50	19–235	41–346	63–367	85–387	107–408
0.75	128–428	150–449	171–469	192–489	213–509
1.00	233–528	254–548	274–567	295–586	315–605
1.25	335–624	355–643	374–661	394–680	413–698
1.50	432–716	451–734	470–752	489–769	507–787
1.75	525–804	544–821	562–838	580–855	597–871
2.00	615–888	632–904	650–920	667–936	684–952
2.25	700–968	717–983	733–999	750–1014	766–1029
2.50	782–1044	798–1059	813–1073	829–1088	844–1102

Table CV1.5. Normal range ($-2SD$ to $+2SD$) for cardiac volume (ml) calculated according to the formula $V = F \times A \times B \times C$, for boys, standing during the examination. The volume is related to body surface area according to Du Bois and Du Bois (1916) (Appendix 1). (After Ghaffarpour et al. 1966)

Body surface area (m²)	—	+ 0.05	+ 0.10	+ 0.15	+ 0.20
0.50	0–366	20–390	45–413	69–437	93–460
0.75	118–483	141–506	165–528	189–551	212–573
1.00	236–596	259–618	282–640	305–662	328–683
1.25	350–705	373–726	395–748	418–769	440–790
1.50	462–811	483–831	505–852	526–872	548–893
1.75	569–913	590–933	611–953	632–972	652–992
2.00	673–1011	693–1031	714–1050	734–1069	754–1088
2.25	773–1106	793–1125	813–1143	832–1162	851–1180
2.50	870–1198	889–1216	908–1233	927–1251	945–1268

References:

Dahlström A, Ringertz H: Normal radiographic heart volume in the neonate. 2. Method of assessment. Pediatr Radiol 1984; 14:288.
Du Bois D, Du Bois EF: Arch Intern Med 1916; 17:863.

CV2   Heart volume in the neonate/weight and age [radiography]

Referenced article:

Dahlström A, Ringertz H: Normal radiographic heart volume in the neonate. 2. Method of assessment. Pediatr Radiol 1984; 14:288.

Background:

Contrary to other standards for measurement of the heart volume in neonates (Lind 1950; Ghaffarpour et al. 1966), the present method takes into account the wide variations that are normally present during the first 48 or 96 hours of life, during which period the ductus arteriosus becomes closed. Three-dimensional methods for calculation of volume are the most accurate, and

Table CV2.1. Normal upper limit (+ 2SD) for cardiac volume (ml). (After Dahlström and Ringertz 1984)

Body weight (kg)	—	+0.1	+0.2	+0.3	+0.4
1st day of life					
1.5	0.1–38.1	1.7–39.8	3.3–41.4	5.0–43.0	6.6–44.6
2.0	8.2–46.3	9.8–47.9	11.5–49.5	13.1–51.1	14.7–52.7
2.5	16.3–54.4	18.0–56.0	19.6–57.6	21.2–59.2	22.8–60.9
3.0	24.5–62.5	26.1–64.1	27.7–65.7	29.3–67.4	31.0–69.0
3.5	32.6–70.6	34.2–72.2	35.8–73.9	37.5–75.5	39.1–77.1
4.0	40.7–78.7	42.3–80.4	43.9–82.0	45.6–83.6	47.2–85.2
4.5	48.8–86.9	50.4–88.5	52.1–90.1	53.7–91.7	55.3–93.3
2nd day of life					
1.5	0.2–34.2	1.6–35.6	3.0–36.9	4.4–38.3	5.8–39.7
2.0	7.2–41.1	8.5–42.5	9.9–43.9	11.3–45.3	12.7–46.7
2.5	14.1–48.0	15.5–49.4	16.9–50.8	18.3–52.2	19.6–53.6
3.0	21.0–55.0	22.4–56.4	23.8–57.8	25.2–59.1	26.6–60.5
3.5	28.0–61.9	29.4–63.3	30.7–64.7	32.1–66.1	33.5–67.5
4.0	34.9–68.9	36.3–70.2	37.7–71.6	39.1–73.0	40.4–74.4
4.5	41.8–75.8	43.2–77.2	44.6–78.6	46.0–79.9	47.4–81.3
3rd–15th day of life					
1.0	5.6–24.7	6.6–25.7	7.6–26.7	8.6–27.7	9.6–28.7
1.5	10.6–29.7	11.6–30.7	12.6–31.7	13.6–32.7	14.6–33.7
2.0	15.6–34.7	16.6–35.7	17.6–36.7	18.6–37.7	19.6–38.7
2.5	20.6–39.7	21.6–40.7	22.6–41.7	23.6–42.7	24.6–43.7
3.0	25.6–44.7	26.6–45.7	27.6–46.7	28.6–47.6	29.6–48.6
3.5	30.5–49.6	31.5–50.6	32.5–51.6	33.5–52.6	34.5–53.6
4.0	35.5–54.6	36.5–55.6	37.5–56.6	38.5–57.6	39.5–58.6
4.5	40.5–59.6	41.5–60.6	42.5–61.6	43.5–62.6	44.5–63.6
5.0	45.5–64.6	46.5–65.6	47.5–66.6	48.5–67.6	49.5–68.6
5.5	50.5–69.6	51.5–70.6	52.5–71.6	53.5–72.6	54.5–73.6

given modern computer aids the procedure is easy to perform and straightforward (Hunt and Williams 1981).

Material:

Chest radiographs in 117 children, aged 0–15 days were studied. All children were, in retrospect, considered clinically normal, and the radiographs revealed normal heart and lungs. The children were radiographed in the supine position with the back or the left side against the cassette. The focus–film distance was 100 cm and the exposures were made at the technologist's estimate of end inspiration.

Method of assessment:

A cardiac silhouette was drawn as close to an ellipse as possible on the AP film (Figure CV1.1). The long axis (A) and the short axis (B) of this ellipse, as well as the greatest horizontal depth of the heart (C) from the lateral film (Figure CV1.1), were used to calculate the heart volume according to the ellipsoid formula: volume $(V) = F \times A \times B \times C$, where the factor F included both the ellipsoid formula constant and the magnification factor. F varied with weight:

below 2.5 kg, $F = 0.421$
for weight 2.5–3.9 kg, $F = 0.439$
for weight above 3.9 kg, $F = 0.453$

It should be observed that for other focus–film distances, F will be different, as is described in the referenced article.

References:

Ghaffarpour R, Ringertz H, Rudhe U, Wallgren G, Röntgenologisk hjärtvolymbestämning hos barn. Läkartidningen 1966; 63:3764 (in Swedish).
Hunt TH, Williams RC: Programmed calculation of cardiac size. AJR 1981; 137:416.
Lind J: Heart volume in normal infants. A roentgenological study. Acta Radiol [Suppl] 1950; 82.

CV3 Cardiothoracic ratio in newborn [radiography]

Referenced article:

Edwards DK, Higgins CB, Gilpin EA: The cardiothoracic ratio in newborn infants. AJR 1981; 136:907.

Background:

The cardiothoracic ratio as measured on AP films is an uncertain measure of the cardiac size, and experienced observations may be better than such measurement. However, it may be of value for radiologists who are relatively inexperienced with infants and it is a simple measure, which is easily understood.

Material:

Chest radiographs in 175 children, aged 0–7 days were studied. In retrospect, the children were clinically considered normal, with no symptoms of lung or heart disease, and the radiographs were normal.

Method of assessment:

The width of the cardiac silhouette was measured on the AP film as the sum of the greatest extent of the cardiac silhouette to the left and the right of the midline of the spine (Figure CV3.1). The thoracic diameters were measured as described in Figure CV3.1, at levels defined in Table CV3.1.

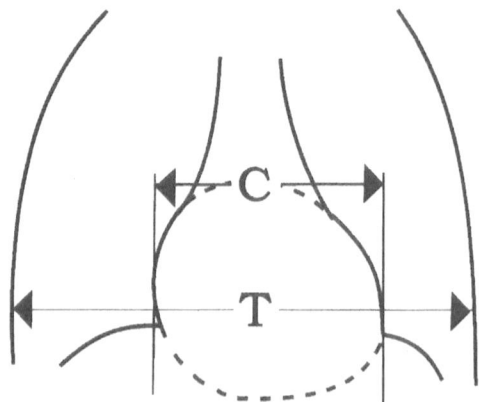

Figure CV3.1. Diameters used for calculation of the cardiothoracic ratio. C, the width of the cardiac silhouette at its greatest extent to the right and left of the spine; T, inner width of bony thorax (measured at different levels, see Table CV3.1). Also, the length of the thoracic spine (T1–T12) was measured. (After Edwards et al. 1981.)

Table CV3.1. Normal ranges (−2SD to +2SD) for four ratios between the maximum width of the cardiac silhouette and the thoracic diameter at different levels in newborns. (After Edwards et al. 1981)

Maximum cardiac width divided by:	Ratio:
1. Inner width of bony thorax at the level of the dome of the right hemidiaphragm	0.458–0.628
2. Inner width of bony thorax at the level of the eighth rib	0.433–0.562
3. Inner width of bony thorax at the widest level	0.427–0.557
4. Length of thoracic spine	0.472–0.641

CV4 Left ventricular end diastolic diameter/weight [sonography]

Referenced article:

Gutgesell HP, Paquet M, Duff DF, McNamara DG: Evaluation of left ventricular size and function by echocardiography. Results in normal children. Circulation 1977; 56:457.

Background:

The size of the left ventricular end diastolic diameter is important for study of cardiac function in children, and may be the most elementary index of the left ventricular function.

Material:

Echocardiograms from 145 normal children (80 boys and 65 girls, aged 1 day–19 years) were studied. For echocardiography transducers of 2.25–5.0 mHz were used, depending on the child's size. Studies were obtained from the third or fourth intercostal space at the left parasternal edge, with the child in the supine position.

Table CV4.1. Normal range (−2SD to +2SD) for sonographically determined left ventricular diameter (mm) related to body weight in kg between 3 and 79 kg. Example: a normal child with a body weight of 23 kg has a 96% probability of having a left ventricular diameter of between 29.4 and 42.2 mm. (After Gutgesell et al. 1977)

Body weight (kg)	−	+ 1	+ 2	+ 3	+ 4
0	–	–	–	10.7–23.5	13.3–26.1
5	15.4–28.2	17.1–29.9	18.5–31.3	19.7–32.5	20.8–33.6
10	21.8–34.6	22.6–35.4	23.5–36.3	24.2–37.0	24.9–37.7
15	25.5–38.3	26.1–38.9	26.7–39.5	27.2–40.0	27.7–40.5
20	28.2–41.0	28.6–41.4	29.0–41.8	29.4–42.2	29.8–42.6
25	30.2–43.0	30.6–43.4	30.9–43.7	31.3–44.1	31.6–44.4
30	31.9–44.7	32.2–45.0	32.5–45.3	32.8–45.6	33.1–45.9
35	33.3–46.1	33.6–46.4	33.8–46.6	34.1–46.9	34.3–47.1
40	34.6–47.4	34.8–47.6	35.0–47.8	35.2–48.0	35.4–48.2
45	35.6–48.4	35.8–48.6	36.0–48.8	36.2–49.0	36.4–49.2
50	36.6–49.4	36.8–49.6	37.0–49.8	37.1–49.9	37.3–50.1
55	37.5–50.3	37.7–50.5	37.8–50.6	38.0–50.8	38.1–50.9
60	38.3–51.1	38.4–51.2	38.6–51.4	38.7–51.5	38.9–51.7
65	39.0–51.8	39.2–52.0	39.3–52.1	39.4–52.2	39.6–52.4
70	39.7–52.5	39.8–52.6	40.0–52.8	40.1–52.9	40.2–53.0
75	40.3–53.1	40.5–53.3	40.6–53.4	40.7–53.5	40.8–53.6

Method of assessment:

The diastolic diameter was measured between the endocardial surfaces of the ventricular septum and the left ventricular posterior wall at the start of the QRS-complex of the electrocardiogram. Normal ranges related to body weight are given in Table CV4.1.

CV5 Diameter of pulmonary veins/height [angiocardiography]

Referenced article:

Robida A: Diameters of pulmonary veins in normal children – an angiocardiographic study. Cardiovasc Intervent Radiol 1990; 12:307.

Background:

Stenosis of the individual pulmonary veins is now surgically correctable. Therefore, knowledge of the normal size is important.

Material:

Cineangiocardiographic films of 27 children without heart disease were studied. The children's heights ranged from 95.5 to 180 cm (mean 128.5 cm).

Method of assessment:

Measurements were obtained in the frontal projection on the levophase of the pulmonary trunk angiograms at the junction of the individual pulmonary veins

Table CV5.1. Normal range ($-$2SD to $+$2SD) for pulmonary vein diameter (mm) in children. A common regression line for all four pulmonary veins has been used. Example: a normal child with the body height 142 cm has a 95% probability of having each of the four pulmonary vein diameters between 10.6 and 12.9 mm. (After Robida 1990)

Body height (cm)	–	+ 1	+ 2	+ 3	+ 4
95	7.5–9.8	7.5–9.9	7.6–9.9	7.7–10.0	7.7–10.1
100	7.8–10.1	7.9–10.2	7.9–10.2	8.0–10.3	8.1–10.4
105	8.1–10.4	8.2–10.5	8.3–10.6	8.3–10.6	8.4–10.7
110	8.5–10.8	8.5–10.8	8.6–10.9	8.7–11.0	8.7–11.0
115	8.8–11.1	8.9–11.2	8.9–11.2	9.0–11.3	9.1–11.4
120	9.1–11.4	9.2–11.5	9.2–11.6	9.3–11.6	9.4–11.7
125	9.4–11.8	9.5–11.8	9.6–11.9	9.6–12.0	9.7–12.0
130	9.8–12.1	9.8–12.1	9.9–12.2	10.0–12.3	10.0–12.3
135	10.1–12.4	10.2–12.5	10.2–12.5	10.3–12.6	10.4–12.7
140	10.4–12.7	10.5–12.8	10.6–12.9	10.6–12.9	10.7–13.0
145	10.8–13.1	10.8–13.1	10.9–13.2	11.0–13.3	11.0–13.3
150	11.1–13.4	11.1–13.5	11.2–13.5	11.3–13.6	11.3–13.7
155	11.4–13.7	11.5–13.8	11.5–13.9	11.6–13.9	11.7–14.0
160	11.7–14.0	11.8–14.1	11.9–14.2	11.9–14.2	12.0–14.3
165	12.1–14.4	12.1–14.4	12.2–14.5	12.3–14.6	12.3–14.6
170	12.4–14.7	12.5–14.8	12.5–14.8	12.6–14.9	12.7–15.0
175	12.7–15.0	12.8–15.1	12.9–15.2	12.9–15.2	13.0–15.3

with the left atrium. For measurement, calipers and a micrometer were used. To eliminate the effect of magnification, the measured size of the intracardiac catheter was used for calibration. Normal ranges related to body weight are given in Table CV5.1.

CV6 Diameter of the right descending pulmonary artery/probability of shunt [radiography]

Referenced article:

Coussement AM, Gooding CA: Objective radiographic assessment of pulmonary vascularity in children. Pediatr Radiol 1973; 109:649.

Background:

When a left-to-right shunt is suspected, evaluation of the width of the pulmonary vessels is important. On the AP radiographs the right descending pulmonary artery may be measured with accuracy. In the present assessment, the width of the right descending pulmonary artery has been compared with the trachea, to eliminate variable factors such as magnification, age and body surface area.

Material:

Chest radiographs from 112 children were studied. None of the children had any disease related to the cardiovascular system.

Method of assessment:

The diameter of the right descending pulmonary artery (RDPA) and of the trachea were measured directly on the frontal chest radiographs. The RDPA was measured at the level where it parallels the right main stem bronchus and crosses the pulmonary vein that drains the right upper lobe (Figure CV6.1). The tracheal diameter was measured just above the impression of the aorta.

The diameters of the RDPA and the trachea were subtracted. The result of this subtraction as an expression of the probability of a shunt being present is given in Table CV6.1.

Table CV6.1. Probability of normality or shunt when the difference between the diameter of the right descending pulmonary artery branch (RDPA) and the trachea is negative, between 0 and 3 mm, or more than 3 mm. The distribution of normal and shunt cases is shown. (After Coussement and Gooding 1973)

Difference	% of normal	% of shunt	Comment
Negative	33	0	No shunt
0 mm	43	10	Prob. 1.7 of shunt
1 mm	14	28	Prob. 14.5 of shunt
2 mm	7	23	Prob. 23.7 of shunt
3 mm	3	15	Prob. 36.1 of shunt
> 3 mm	0	24	Shunt (24%)
Sum	100	100	

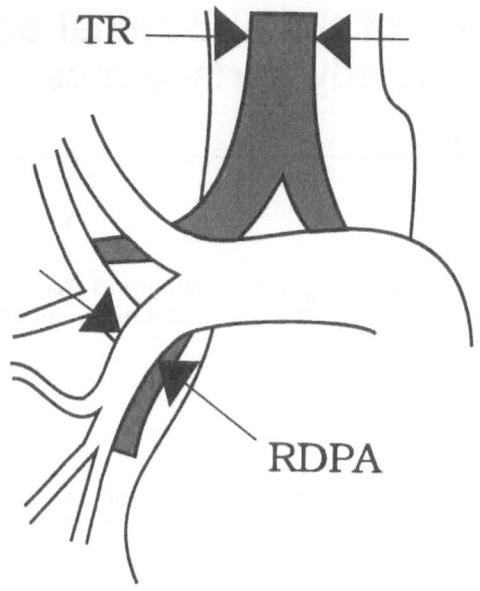

Figure CV6.1. Sites for measurement of the pulmonary artery (RDPA) and the trachea (TR). (After Coussement and Gooding 1973.)

CV7 Diameter of the abdominal aorta at different levels/body surface area [radiography]

Referenced article:

Taber P, Korobkin MT, Gooding CA, Palubinskas AJ, Neuhauser EBD: Growth of the abdominal aorta and renal arteries in childhood. Radiology 1972; 102:129.

Table CV7.1. Normal range (−2SD to +2SD) of the aortic diameter for children of both sexes in relation to body surface area. The ranges are given for three different levels of the aorta: at the level of 11th thoracic vertebral body, at the renal artery, and just above the bifurcation. (After Taber et al. 1972)

Body surface area (m²)	Aortic diameter (mm)		
	T11	Renal artery	Bifurcation
0.20	4.0–10.0	2.4–9.6	1.6–7.4
0.25	4.4–10.4	2.8–9.9	1.9–7.8
0.30	4.8–10.8	3.2–10.3	2.3–8.1
0.35	5.2–11.2	3.5–10.7	2.7–8.5
0.40	5.6–11.6	3.9–11.0	3.1–8.9
0.45	5.9–12.0	4.2–11.4	3.5–9.3
0.50	6.3–12.4	4.6–11.7	3.9–9.7
0.55	6.7–12.7	4.9–12.1	4.2–10.0
0.60	7.1–13.1	5.3–12.4	4.6–10.4
0.65	7.5–13.5	5.7–12.8	5.0–10.8
0.70	7.9–13.9	6.0–13.2	5.4–11.2
0.75	8.3–14.3	6.4–13.5	5.8–11.6
0.80	8.7–14.7	6.7–13.9	6.1–12.0
0.85	9.0–15.1	7.1–14.2	6.5–12.3
0.90	9.4–15.5	7.4–14.6	6.9–12.7
0.95	9.8–15.8	7.8–14.9	7.3–13.1
1.00	10.2–16.2	8.2–15.3	7.7–13.5
1.05	10.6–16.6	8.5–15.7	8.1–13.9
1.10	11.0–17.0	8.9–16.0	8.4–14.2
1.15	11.4–17.4	9.2–16.4	8.8–14.6
1.20	11.8–17.8	9.6–16.7	9.2–15.0
1.25	12.1–18.2	9.9–17.1	9.6–15.4
1.30	12.5–18.6	10.3–17.4	10.0–15.8
1.35	12.9–18.9	10.7–17.8	10.3–16.2
1.40	13.3–19.3	11.0–18.2	10.7–16.5
1.45	13.7–19.7	11.4–18.5	11.1–16.9
1.50	14.1–20.1	11.7–18.9	11.5–17.3

Background:

Hypoplasia of the abdominal aorta is uncommon, but may appear in a variety of pathological conditions. In many of these, only the intraluminal diameter is diminished, while the external calibre may be normal. Measurement of the lumen is therefore essential.

Material:

Unselected abdominal aortograms of 45 patients, aged 1 day–15 years were studied. Focus–film distance was 40 inches (101.6 cm).

Method of assessment:

The diameter of the aorta (Table CV7.1) was measured at

A: The level of the pedicles of the 11th thoracic vertebra
B: Just above the renal arteries
C: At the aortic bifurcation

The diameter of the aorta was related to body surface area (Du Bois and Du Bois 1916) (see Appendix I).

Reference:

Du Bois D, Du Bois EF: Arch Intern Med 1916; 17:863.

SECTION 8
The Abdomen

AB1   Liver size/height/age [radiography]

Referenced article:

Deligeorgis D, Yannakos D, Doxiadis S: Normal size of liver in infancy and childhood. X-ray study. Arch Dis Child 1973; 48:790.

Background:

An estimate of the liver size may be obtained at radiography, even if both ultrasound and scintigraphy offer more accurate information.

Material:

AP radiographs of the abdomen from 350 normal children, aged neonate–15 years were studied. The child was supine, with the central beam towards the liver with focus–film distance of 140 cm.

Method of assessment:

A horizontal line was drawn tangential to the uppermost region of the liver, just below the dome of the diaphragm and another horizontal line was drawn parallel to the first, tangential to the lowest part of the liver. The vertical distance between the two lines was defined as the vertical axis.

Normal ranges for the vertical axis of the liver in relation to height and age are given in Tables AB1.1 and AB1.2 respectively.

Table AB1.1. Normal range (−2SD to +2SD) for the vertical axis of the liver in mm in relation to body height of children between 0 and 15 years of age and of both sexes. The normal range is given in steps of 2 cm of body height between 46 and 178 cm. For example, the normal range for the vertical axis of the liver for a child 126 cm tall is 116–167 mm. (After Deligeorgis et al. 1973)

Height (cm)	−	+2	+4	+6	+8
40				43–94	45–96
50	47–98	49–100	51–102	52–103	54–105
60	56–107	58–109	60–111	61–112	63–114
70	65–116	67–118	69–120	71–122	72–123
80	74–125	76–127	78–129	80–131	81–132
90	83–134	85–136	87–138	89–140	90–141
100	92–143	94–145	96–147	98–149	99–150
110	101–152	103–154	105–156	107–158	108–159
120	110–161	112–163	114–165	116–167	118–169
130	119–170	121–172	123–174	125–176	127–178
140	128–179	130–181	132–183	134–185	136–187
150	137–188	139–190	141–192	143–194	145–196
160	146–197	148–199	150–201	152–203	154–205
170	155–206	157–208	159–210	161–212	163–214

Table AB1.2. Normal range (−2SD to +2SD) for the vertical axis of the liver in mm in relation to age in children of both sexes between 0 and 15.5 years of age. (After Deligeorgis et al. 1973)

Age (years)	Height (mm)	Age (years)	Height (mm)	Age (years)	Height (mm)	Age (years)	Height (mm)
0.0	57–84	0.5	69–110	1.0	74–121	1.5	77–130
2.0	80–137	2.5	83–143	3.0	86–149	3.5	88–154
4.0	90–159	4.5	92–164	5.0	94–168	5.5	96–172
6.0	97–176	6.5	99–180	7.0	100–183	7.5	102–187
8.0	103–190	8.5	105–194	9.0	106–197	9.5	108–200
10.0	109–203	10.5	110–206	11.0	111–209	11.5	113–211
12.0	114–214	12.5	115–217	13.0	116–220	13.5	117–222
14.0	118–225	14.5	120–227	15.0	121–230	15.5	122–232

AB2   Size of liver and spleen/age and weight [scintigraphy]

Referenced article:

Markisz JA, Treves ST, Davis RT: Normal hepatic and splenic size in children: scintigraphic determination. Pediatr Radiol 1987; 17:273.

Background:

Determination of hepatomegaly and splenomegaly should be an integral part of the analysis of liver/spleen scintigraphy.

Material:

Scintigraphies from 131 studies on 116 patients (71 boys, 45 girls), without any signs of liver or spleen disease were used.

The patients had an i.v. injection of ^{99m}Tc sulphur-colloid (0.04 mCi/kg with a 0.5 mCi minimum and 3.0 mCi maximum). Multiple projections of the liver and spleen were obtained using a parallel hole collimator. Anterior and right lateral views were used for obtaining measurements of the liver and the posterior view was used for splenic values.

Method of assessment:

Measurements of the liver were obtained as follows:

1. Horizontal parallel lines were drawn through the most superior and most inferior aspects of the liver as viewed in the anterior projection and the perpendicular distance between them was taken as the vertical span or height (A) (Figure AB2.1).
2. Vertical parallel lines were drawn at the extreme right and left borders of the liver on the anterior projection and the perpendicular distance between them was designated as the horizontal span or width (B) (Figure AB2.1).

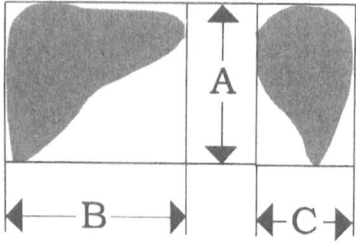

Figure AB2.1. Diameters measured for calculation of liver size (see text). (After Markisz et al. 1978.)

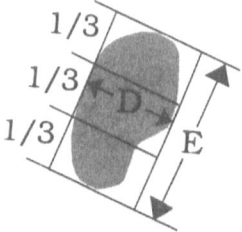

Figure AB2.2. Diameters measured for calculation of spleen size (see text). (After Markisz et al. 1978.)

Table AB2.1. Normal range (−2SD to +2SD) for scintigraphically determined normal hepatic and splenic volume in children related to body weight from 10 to 70 kg. (After Markisz et al. 1987)

Body weight (kg)	Liver volume (cm³)	Spleen volume (cm³)
10	160– 811	0–107
12	226– 877	0–113
14	292– 943	0–119
16	358–1009	0–125
18	424–1075	0–131
20	490–1141	3–137
22	556–1207	9–143
24	622–1273	15–149
26	688–1339	21–155
28	754–1405	27–161
30	820–1471	33–166
32	886–1537	39–172
34	952–1603	45–178
36	1018–1669	51–184
38	1084–1735	57–190
40	1150–1801	63–196
42	1216–1867	69–202
44	1282–1933	75–208
46	1348–1998	81–214
48	1414–2064	87–220
50	1480–2130	93–226
52	1546–2196	99–232
54	1612–2262	105–238
56	1677–2328	111–244
58	1743–2394	117–250
60	1809–2460	123–256
62	1875–2526	129–262
64	1941–2592	135–268
66	2007–2658	141–274
68	2073–2724	146–280
70	2139–2790	152–286

3. Vertical lines were drawn through the most anterior and posterior aspects of the liver on the right lateral view and the perpendicular distance between them was designated as the right lateral dimension or depth (C) (Figure AB2.1).

Measurements of the spleen were obtained using the posterior projection. The longest linear distance between the two poles was designated as the major axis (E) (Figure AB2.2) and the greatest linear distance perpendicular to the major axis in the middle third of the spleen was called the minor axis (D) (Figure AB2.2).

The liver volume V_L was calculated according to the formula

$$V_L = \frac{\pi}{8} \cdot ABC$$

and the volume of the spleen, V_S, was calculated according to the formula

$$V_S = \frac{\pi}{8} \cdot ED^2$$

Normal ranges for hepatic and splenic volume are given in Table AB2.1.

AB3 Size of liver and spleen/body weight and height [ultrasound]

Referenced article:

Dittrich M, Milde S, Dinkel E, Baumann W, Weitzel D: Sonographic biometry of liver and spleen size in childhood. Pediatr Radiol 1983; 13:206.

Background:

For evaluation of size of the liver and spleen, ultrasound is easy to use and has few disadvantages.

Material:

Ultrasound examinations in 194 children, aged 10 days–17.6 years were studied. The children had no signs of liver or spleen disease.

The examinations were performed with a real-time parallel scanner or a real-time sector scanner, 3.5 MHz. For measurements of liver size, the patients were investigated in the supine position, and for spleen size in the right-recumbent position.

Method of assessment:

The craniocaudal liver extension was measured in three standardised planes, as shown in Figure AB3.1. On the basis of external orientation lines, the section planes were defined in terms of the longitudinal axis of the body taking into account the largest optical organ section area and topographical landmarks. The section level in the anterior axillary line (AAL) was fixed by the optically largest section area of the liver and the section level in the medioclavicular line (MCL) by simultaneous visualisation of the right kidney. The perpendicular section plane in the sternal line (STL) was determined by simultaneous demonstration of the abdominal aorta. The extension in the anterior axillary

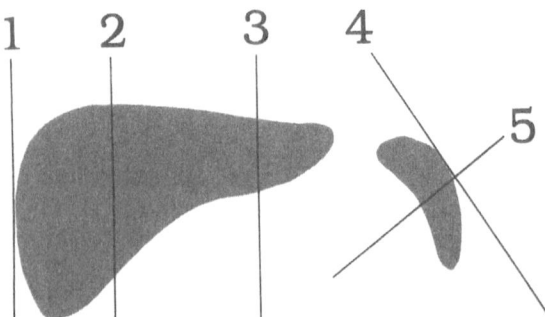

Figure AB3.1. Section planes for evaluation of liver and spleen size. 1, Anterior axillary line; 2, medioclavicular line; 3, sternal line; 4, longitudinal section; 5, transverse section. (After Dittrich et al. 1983.)

line (AAL), in the medioclavicular line (MCL), and in the sternal line (STL) was used to calculate the index of liver size (ILS):

$$ILS = \frac{\pi}{3 \cdot 4} (AAL^2 + MCL^2 + STL^2)$$

For spleen size, the maximum extent was measured as length (L) and depth (D_L) or breadth (B) and depth (D_B), in the longitudinal and transverse planes (Figure AB3.1). The spleen volume (SV) was calculated according to the formula for an ellipsoid:

$$SV = L\,B\,\frac{D_L + D_B}{2}\,0.523\ cm^3$$

Normal ranges of liver index and spleen volume are given in Table AB3.1.

Table AB3.1. Normal ranges (−2SD to +2SD) for the liver index determined by ultrasonic examinations as described in the text and splenic volume, both related to body heights. (After Dittrich et al. 1983)

Body height (cm)	Liver index (cm²)	Spleen size (cm³)
55	5.7–33.6	0.0–30.4
60	8.1–36.7	0.0–33.8
65	10.4–39.9	0.0–37.2
70	12.7–43.0	1.0–40.7
75	15.1–46.1	3.0–44.1
80	17.4–49.2	5.0–47.5
85	19.7–52.4	6.9–50.9
90	22.1–55.5	8.9–54.3
95	24.4–58.6	10.9–57.7
100	26.7–61.7	12.8–61.1
105	29.1–64.9	14.8–64.5
110	31.4–68.0	16.7–67.9
115	33.7–71.1	18.7–71.4
120	36.1–74.2	20.7–74.8
125	38.4–77.4	22.6–78.2
130	40.7–80.5	24.6–81.6
135	43.1–83.6	26.6–85.0
140	45.4–86.7	28.5–88.4
145	47.7–89.8	30.5–91.8
150	50.0–93.0	32.5–95.2
155	52.4–96.1	34.4–98.6
160	54.7–99.2	36.4–102.1
165	57.0–102.3	38.4–105.5
170	59.4–105.5	40.3–108.9

AB4 Size of gallbladder and biliary tract [ultrasound]

Referenced article:

McGahan JP, Phillips HE, Cox KL: Sonography of the normal pediatric gallbladder and biliary tract. Radiology 1982; 14:873.

Background:

Normal parameters of the pediatric gallbladder and biliary tract may be of value especially in the ultrasonic evaluation of cholecystitis.

Material:

A total of 51 children, aged 1 month–16 years, with no history or signs of disease affecting the upper abdomen were studied. Younger patients had fasted for three hours, older patients for eight hours. The examinations were performed with a digital grey-scale scanner or a real-time scanner, 3.5–5.0 MHz.

Method of measurement:

The following measurements were performed: maximum length and AP diameter of the gallbladder, as measured on parasagittal scans, as well as width (coronal size) as obtained with cross-sectional scans (Table AB4.1). Slightly oblique scans were also obtained in order to determine the greatest width,

Table AB4.1. Normal ranges (−2SD to +2SD) for the AP and coronal diameter as well as length of the gallbladder and the diameter of the right portal vein (mm). (After McGahan et al. 1982)

Age (years)	AP diameter (mm)	Coronal diameter (mm)	Length (mm)	Right portal vein (mm)
0	5.7– 9.7	5.1–18.1	11.4–25.2	2.1– 4.0
1	7.8–15.5	7.6–22.9	19.8–40.0	3.0– 5.6
2	8.7–17.9	8.6–24.9	23.2–46.1	3.4– 6.3
3	9.3–19.8	9.3–26.5	25.8–50.8	3.7– 6.8
4	9.9–21.3	10.0–27.7	28.1–54.7	4.0– 7.3
5	10.4–22.7	10.5–28.9	30.0–58.2	4.2– 7.7
6	10.8–23.9	11.1–29.9	31.8–61.3	4.4– 8.0
7	11.3–25.1	11.5–30.9	33.4–64.2	4.6– 8.4
8	11.6–26.1	12.0–31.7	35.0–66.9	4.8– 8.7
9	12.0–27.1	12.4–32.6	36.4–69.5	5.0– 9.0
10	12.4–28.1	12.8–33.3	37.7–71.9	5.1– 9.2
11	12.7–29.0	13.2–34.1	39.0–74.1	5.3– 9.5
12	13.0–29.8	13.5–34.8	40.3–76.3	5.4– 9.7
13	13.3–30.6	13.9–35.5	41.4–78.4	5.5–10.0
14	13.6–31.4	14.2–36.1	42.6–80.4	5.7–10.2
15	13.9–32.2	14.5–36.8	43.7–82.3	5.8–10.4

Table AB4.2. Gallbladder wall thickness and the common hepatic duct diameter. There was no significant change with age; the estimated normal range (−2SD to +2SD) is thus given for all ages. (After McGahan et al. 1982)

Gallbladder wall thickness	1.0–3.0 mm
Common hepatic duct diameter	1.0–4.0 mm

length and AP diameter. All measurements were made intraluminally. Also, the wall thickness and the distance between the inner walls of the common hepatic duct were measured (Table AB4.2), as was the diameter of the right portal vein on parasagittal scans.

AB5 Width of common bile duct/age [cholangiography]

Referenced article:

Witcombe JB, Cremin BJ: The width of the common bile duct in childhood. Pediatr Radiol 1978; 7:147.

Background:

Dilatation of the common bile duct is a useful cholangiographic sign of biliary obstruction. However, today the size of the biliary tree is most easily assessed using ultrasound.

Material:

Cholangiographic examinations in 85 children (41 boys, 44 girls), aged 1–14 years were used. The examinations were performed using 20 ml of 50% meglumine iodipamide, as direct injection or drip infusion. Radiographs were taken in a 15° prone oblique position, with focus–film distance of 100 cm.

Method of assessment:

The widest transverse diameter of the common bile duct was measured. Measurements were avoided within 5 mm of the origin of the common bile duct. No correction was made for magnification.

Normal ranges are given in Table AB5.1.

Table AB5.1. Normal range (−2SD to +2SD) for the width of the common bile duct as estimated by cholangiography related to age between 2 and 13.5 years. (After Witcombe and Cremin 1978)

Age (years)	Width (mm)	Age (years)	Width (mm)	Age (years)	Width (mm)	Age (years)	Width (mm)
2.0	0.6–4.5	2.5	0.7–4.6	3.0	0.8–4.7	3.5	0.9–4.8
4.0	1.0–4.9	4.5	1.2–5.0	5.0	1.3–5.1	5.5	1.4–5.2
6.0	1.5–5.3	6.5	1.6–5.4	7.0	1.7–5.6	7.5	1.8–5.7
8.0	1.9–5.8	8.5	2.0–5.9	9.0	2.1–6.0	9.5	2.3–6.1
10.0	2.4–6.2	10.5	2.5–6.3	11.0	2.6–6.4	11.5	2.7–6.5
12.0	2.8–6.6	12.5	2.9–6.8	13.0	3.0–6.9	13.5	3.1–7.0

AB6 Muscle dimensions of the pylorus [ultrasound]

Referenced article:

Kofoed PEL, Höst A, Elle B, Larssen C: Hypertrophic pyloric stenosis: determination of muscle dimensions by ultrasound. Br J Radiol 1988; 61:19.

Background:

Hypertrophic pyloric stenosis may today be diagnosed using ultrasound. The ultrasound diagnosis depends on measurements of the pyloric diameter, the pyloric length, and the muscle thickness.

Material:

Determinations were carried out on 34 normal controls, aged 3–135 days (mean: 39.2 days). The ultrasound examination was performed using a real-time sector scanner with a 5 MHz transducer.

Method of assessment:

The pyloric muscle was measured for diameter, length and wall thickness (Table AB6.1).

Table AB6.1. Normal range ($-2SD$ to $+2SD$) for ultrasonographic measurements of pyloric length, diameter, and thickness in normal children aged between 3 and 135 days. The corresponding total values for less well-defined normal materials are given in parentheses. (After Kofoed et al. 1988)

Pyloric length (mm)	6.4–19.6	(4.8–15.2)[a]
Pyloric diameter (mm)	4.1–12.9	(5.6–12.0)[a]
Wall thickness (mm)	1.5–5.5	(1.1–3.2)[b]

[a] From Stunden et al. (1986) and Westra et al. (1989).
[b] From Blumhagen and Noble (1983), Gomes and Menanteau (1983) and Stunden et al. (1986) in addition to the referenced material.

References:

Blumhagen JD, Noble HGS: Muscle thickness in hypertrophic pyloric stenosis: sonographic determination. AJR 1983; 140:221–223.
Gomes H, Menanteau B: Aspects échographiques du pylore normal et hypertrophie (Sonography of normal and hypertrophic pylorus). Ann Radiol 1983; 26:154–160.
Stunden RJ, LeQuesne GW, Little KET: The improved ultrasound diagnosis of hypertrophic pyloric stenosis. Pediatr Radiol 1986; 16:200–205.
Westra SJ, De Groot CJ, Smits NJ, Staalman CR: Hypertrophic pyloric stenosis: use of the pyloric volume measurement in early US diagnosis. Radiology 1989; 172:615–619.

AB7   Diameter of gas filled bowel loops in infants [radiography]

Referenced article:

Edwards DK: Size of gas-filled bowel loops in infants. AJR 1980; 135:331.

Background:

Gaseous distension of bowel loops is a frequent early radiographic manifestation of necrotising enterocolitis. There is a correlation between the degree of distension and the severity of the disease. Numerical standards for the size of bowel loops may facilitate diagnosis of abnormal dilatation and may serve as a basis for a numerical description of the degree of dilatation.

Material:

AP radiographs of the abdomen from 355 infants who had no sign or suspicion of abdominal disease were studied. Almost all the examinations had been performed to establish umbilical catheter position in patients with lung disease. The patients were supine, with a film–focus distance of 102 cm. No correction was made for magnification.

Table AB7.1. Normal range (−2SD to +2SD) for maximum bowel loop width (mm) in the newborn related to the width of the body of L1, the width between the pedicles of L1, and the height of L1 and L2 including the intervertebral space. As an example a normal child with the latter measurement equal to 13 mm has a 96% probability of a maximum bowel width between 5.2 and 10.8 mm. (After Edwards 1980)

Vertebral measurement (mm)	Width L1 body	Width L1 ped	Height L1–L2
5	2.8– 5.3	1.8– 4.0	2.0– 4.2
6	3.4– 6.3	2.2– 4.7	2.4– 5.0
7	3.9– 7.3	2.5– 5.5	2.8– 5.8
8	4.5– 8.4	2.9– 6.3	3.2– 6.6
9	5.0– 9.5	3.2– 7.1	3.6– 7.5
10	5.6–10.5	3.6– 7.9	4.0– 8.3
11	6.2–11.5	4.0– 8.7	4.4– 9.1
12	6.7–12.6	4.3– 9.5	4.8–10.0
13	7.3–13.7	4.7–10.3	5.2–10.8
14	7.8–14.7	5.0–11.1	5.6–11.6
15	8.4–15.7	5.4–11.9	6.0–12.5
16	9.0–16.8	5.8–12.6	6.4–13.3
17	9.5–17.8	6.1–13.4	6.8–14.1
18	10.1–18.9	6.5–14.2	7.2–14.9
19	10.6–19.9	6.8–15.0	7.6–15.8
20	11.2–21.0	7.2–15.8	8.0–16.6

Method of assessment:

The largest gas filled loop was identified and its diameter (B) was measured with calipers. No attempt was made to distinguish large from small bowel.

To obtain a ratio the following measurements were performed on the lumbar spine:

- The width of the first lumbar vertebral body (V1).
- The distance between the outer edges of the pedicles of the first lumbar vertebral body (V2).
- The total height of the vertebral bodies L1 and L2, including the disc space (V3). This measurement is the easiest to perform, and most reproducible.

Normal ranges for these ratios are given in Table AB7.1.

AB8 Diameter of small bowel/age [radiography]

Referenced article:

Haworth EM, Hodson CJ, Joyce CRB, Pringle EM, Solimano G, Young WF: Radiological measurement of small bowel calibre in normal subjects according to age. Clin Radiol 1967; 18:417.

Background:

Measurement of small bowel diameter may be of value in alimentary disturbances like the coeliac syndrome or gluten enteropathy.

Material:

AP radiographs of the abdomen of 61 infants, aged 9 months to 13.5 years, who had had a non-flocculating barium meal were studied. The children were encouraged to lie on their right side after the meal and the examination was performed 30–45 minutes later. The focus–film distance was 36 inches (91.4 cm) and there was no correction made for the magnification.

Method of measurement:

Three segments of the jejunum that had clearly defined margins and were of approximately uniform calibre with the rest of the bowel were selected. The average of the three measurements was calculated and used as the result (Table AB8.1).

Table AB8.1. Normal range ($-2SD$ to $+2SD$) for the diameter of the jejunum related to age between 1 and 15 years for both sexes. The diameter is measured as the average of three normal loops. (After Haworth et al. 1967)

Age (years)	Jejunal diameter (mm)	Age (years)	Jejunal diameter (mm)	Age (years)	Jejunal diameter (mm)
1	11.4–15.8	6	17.0–21.4	11	20.4–24.8
2	13.0–17.4	7	17.8–22.2	12	21.0–25.4
3	14.3–18.7	8	18.5–22.9	13	21.5–25.9
4	15.3–19.7	9	19.2–23.6	14	22.1–26.5
5	16.2–20.6	10	19.8–24.2	15	22.6–27.0

AB9   Retrorectal soft tissue space [radiography]

Referenced article:

Eklöf O, Gierup J: The retrorectal soft tissue space in children: normal variations and appearances in granulomatous colitis. AJR 1970; 108:624.

Background:

In inflammatory disease of the large bowel, the retrorectal soft tissues may be thickened. This can be evaluated on a colon examination.

Material:

Measurements were made on radiographs from 160 children (85 boys and 75 girls, aged 1–15 years) who had barium enema examination of the colon, but who had no signs of inflammatory disease. The radiograph was obtained as a true lateral projection during filling of the large bowel.

Method of assessment:

The shortest distance between the anterior surface of the sacrum and the posterior rectal wall was measured (Table AB9.1). In most cases, this was found at the level of the third or fourth sacral segment.

Table AB9.1 Normal range (−2SD to +2SD) for the shortest retrorectal distance to the sacrum as a measure of retrorectal soft tissue thickness for children of both sexes between 1 and 15 years of age. (After Eklöf and Gierup 1970)

Retrorectal distance	1.3–5.1mm

SECTION 9
The Urinary Tract

UT1 Renal length/L1–L3 [radiography]
Renal parenchymal area/L1–L3 [radiography]
Renal parenchymal thickness/L1–L3 [radiography]

Referenced article:

Claësson I, Jacobsson B, Olsson T, Ringertz H: Assessment of renal parenchymal thickness in normal children. Acta Radiol [Diagn] 1981; 22:305.

Background:

A large number of papers have been published concerning the normal radiological correlation between renal length and a lumbar spine segment (Currarino 1965; Eklöf and Ringertz 1976a, b; Klare et al. 1980). To use the lumbar segment L1–L3 including the intervertebral spaces as reference has the advantage that this segment is always seen on the IVP film. It also means that magnification factors are irrelevant as all structures measured are located in the same plane.

The renal length measurements are mainly intended for screening purposes whereas the other measurements are more time-consuming and intended for follow-up and pathological cases. The renal parenchymal area is a good overall estimate of renal function (Aperia et al. 1978; Jorulf et al. 1978). The parenchymal thickness values are intended for pathological cases with suspected early scarring.

Material:

Claësson et al. (1981) studied urographic films obtained in the supine position in 149 children, aged 1 week–16 years. The kidneys and the lumbar spine were clinically and radiologically normal. Cases with duplications of the upper urinary tract were excluded. A total of 49 of the children had L1–L3 distances between 2.5 and 5.0 cm and were used for special calculations of renal length and parenchymal area for this subgroup.

Method of assessment:

The L1–L3 distance was measured from the upper border of L1 to the lower border of L3 including the intervertebral spaces between by the vertebrae L1 to L3. The length of the kidney was defined as the distance between the two poles along the long axis of the kidney (Figure UT1.1) (Table UT1.1).

The parenchymal area was measured planimetrically or computerised with a digitiser. The total renal area projected on an AP film was reduced with the renal pelvic area including all calyces (Table UT1.2).

Measurements of the parenchymal thickness (Figure UT1.2) were performed at the upper and lower poles (Table UT1.3). The upper and lower measurements were made from the papillary tip of the calyx closest to the pole parallel to the long axis out to the renal outline.

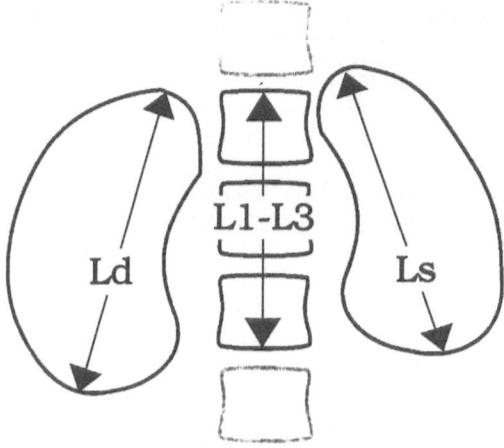

Figure UT1.1. The length of the kidney and the L1–L3 distance. Ld and Ls are the length of the right and left kidney, respectively, measured along the long axis of the kidney; L1–L3 is the L1–L3 distance, including the intervertebral spaces.

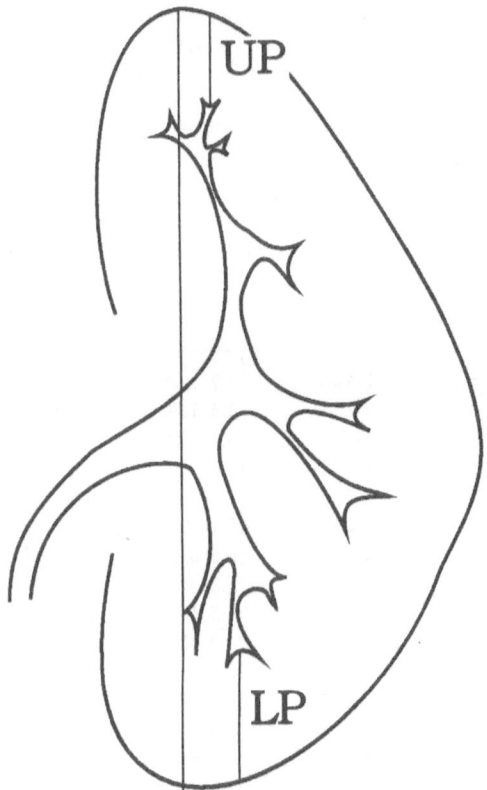

Figure UT1.2. The parenchymal thickness. UP and LP are the upper and lower pole thicknesses, measured from the papillary tip of the calyx closest to the tip to the renal outline, parallel with the long axis of the kidney. (After Claësson et al. 1981.)

Table UT1.1. Normal range (−2SD to +2SD) for renal length (cm) in children up to 15 years related to the length of the lumbar segment L1–L3 including the intervertebral spaces. As an example a child with L1–L3 = 7.3 cm has a 96% probability of having a renal length between 8.3 and 11.1 cm. (After Claësson et al. 1981)

L1–L3 (cm)	–	+ 0.1	+ 0.2	+ 0.3	+ 0.4
2.5	3.7– 5.5	3.8– 5.6	3.9– 5.7	4.1– 5.9	4.2– 6.0
3.0	4.3– 6.1	4.4– 6.2	4.6– 6.4	4.7– 6.5	4.8– 6.6
3.5	4.9– 6.7	5.1– 6.9	5.2– 7.0	5.3– 7.1	5.4– 7.2
4.0	5.5– 7.4	5.5– 7.5	5.6– 7.6	5.7– 7.7	5.8– 7.9
4.5	5.9– 8.0	5.9– 8.1	6.0– 8.2	6.1– 8.4	6.2– 8.5
5.0	6.2– 8.6	6.3– 8.7	6.4– 8.8	6.5– 9.0	6.5– 9.1
5.5	6.6– 9.2	6.7– 9.3	6.7– 9.5	6.8– 9.6	6.9– 9.7
6.0	7.0– 9.8	7.1– 9.9	7.2–10.0	7.3–10.1	7.4–10.2
6.5	7.5–10.3	7.6–10.4	7.7–10.5	7.8–10.6	7.9–10.7
7.0	8.0–10.8	8.1–10.9	8.2–11.0	8.3–11.1	8.4–11.1
7.5	8.5–11.2	8.6–11.3	8.7–11.4	8.8–11.5	8.9–11.6
8.0	9.0–11.7	9.1–11.8	9.2–11.9	9.3–12.0	9.4–12.1
8.5	9.5–12.2	9.6–12.3	9.7–12.4	9.8–12.5	9.9–12.6
9.0	10.0–12.7	10.1–12.8	10.2–12.9	10.3–13.0	10.4–13.1
9.5	10.5–13.2	10.6–13.3	10.7–13.4	10.8–13.5	10.9–13.6
10.0	11.0–13.7	11.1–13.8	11.2–13.9	11.3–14.0	11.4–14.1
10.5	11.5–14.2	11.6–14.3	11.7–14.4	11.8–14.5	11.9–14.6
11.0	12.0–14.7	12.1–14.8	12.2–14.9	12.3–15.0	12.4–15.1

Table UT1.2. Normal range (−2SD to +2SD) for renal area (cm^2) in children up to 15 years related to the length of the lumbar segment L1–L3 including the intervertebral spaces. As an example a child with L1–L3 = 8.3 cm has a 96% probability of having a renal area between 30.2 and 49.5 cm^2. (After Claësson et al. 1981)

L1–L3 (cm)	–	+ 0.1	+ 0.2	+ 0.3	+ 0.4
2.5	2.6–11.1	3.1–11.7	3.7–12.1	4.2–12.8	4.8–13.3
3.0	5.3–13.8	5.9–14.4	6.4–14.9	6.9–15.5	7.5–16.0
3.5	8.0–16.6	8.6–17.1	9.1–17.6	9.7–18.2	10.2–18.7
4.0	10.7–19.3	11.1–20.2	11.4–21.1	11.8–21.9	12.2–22.7
4.5	12.5–23.5	12.9–24.3	13.3–25.1	13.7–26.0	14.0–26.8
5.0	14.4–27.6	14.7–28.4	15.1–29.2	15.5–30.0	15.8–30.8
5.5	16.2–31.6	16.6–32.4	16.9–33.2	17.3–34.0	17.6–34.8
6.0	17.9–35.7	18.2–36.4	18.8–37.0	19.3–37.6	19.8–38.2
6.5	20.4–38.8	20.9–39.4	21.5–40.0	22.0–40.6	22.6–41.2
7.0	23.1–41.8	23.6–42.4	24.2–43.0	24.7–43.6	25.3–44.2
7.5	25.8–44.8	26.4–45.4	26.9–46.0	27.4–46.6	28.0–47.2
8.0	28.5–47.7	29.1–48.3	29.6–48.9	30.2–49.5	30.7–50.1
8.5	31.2–50.7	31.7–51.3	32.3–51.9	32.9–52.5	33.4–53.1
9.0	34.0–53.7	34.5–54.3	35.0–54.9	35.6–55.5	36.1–56.1
9.5	36.7–56.7	37.2–57.3	37.8–57.9	38.3–58.5	38.8–59.1
10.0	39.4–59.7	39.9–60.3	40.5–60.9	41.0–61.5	41.6–62.1
10.5	42.1–62.7	42.6–63.3	43.2–63.9	43.7–64.5	44.3–65.1

Table UT1.3. Normal range (−2SD to +2SD) for parenchymal thickness of the upper (top) and lower pole (bottom) of the kidney. Values are adapted to boys and girls. As an example a normal child with a L1–L3 distance of 103 mm has a 96% probability of having an upper pole parenchymal thickness of 25.9–38.0 mm and a 96% probability of a lower pole between 26.8 and 39.1 mm. (After Claësson et al. 1981)

L1–L3 (mm)	−	+ 1	+ 2	+ 3	+ 4
Upper pole					
50	14.3–26.3	14.5–26.6	14.7–26.8	15.0–27.0	15.2–27.2
55	15.4–27.4	15.6–27.7	15.8–27.9	16.1–28.1	16.3–28.3
60	16.5–28.5	16.7–28.8	16.9–29.0	17.2–29.2	17.4–29.4
65	17.6–29.6	17.8–29.9	18.0–30.1	18.3–30.3	18.5–30.5
70	18.7–30.7	18.9–30.9	19.1–31.2	19.3–31.4	19.6–31.6
75	19.8–31.8	20.0–32.0	20.2–32.3	20.4–32.5	20.7–32.7
80	20.9–32.9	21.1–33.1	21.3–33.4	21.5–33.6	21.8–33.8
85	22.0–34.0	22.2–34.2	22.4–34.5	22.6–34.7	22.9–34.9
90	23.1–35.1	23.3–35.3	23.5–35.5	23.7–35.8	23.9–36.0
95	24.2–36.2	24.4–36.4	24.6–36.6	24.8–36.9	25.0–37.1
100	25.3–37.3	25.5–37.5	25.7–37.7	25.9–38.0	26.1–38.2
105	26.4–38.4	26.6–38.6	26.8–38.8	27.0–39.1	27.2–39.3
110	27.5–39.5	27.7–39.7	27.9–39.9	28.1–40.1	28.3–40.4
115	28.5–40.6	28.8–40.8	29.0–41.0	29.2–41.2	29.4–41.5
Lower pole					
50	14.3–26.6	14.5–26.8	14.8–27.1	15.0–27.3	15.2–27.5
55	15.5–27.8	15.7–28.0	16.0–28.2	16.2–28.5	16.4–28.7
60	16.7–28.9	16.9–29.2	17.1–29.4	17.4–29.7	17.6–29.9
65	17.8–30.1	18.1–30.4	18.3–30.6	18.6–30.8	18.8–31.1
70	19.0–31.3	19.3–31.5	19.5–31.8	19.7–32.0	20.0–32.2
75	20.2–32.5	20.4–32.7	20.7–33.0	20.9–33.2	21.1–33.4
80	21.4–33.7	21.6–33.9	21.9–34.1	22.1–34.4	22.3–34.6
85	22.6–34.8	22.8–35.1	23.0–35.3	23.3–35.6	23.5–35.8
90	23.7–36.0	24.0–36.3	24.2–36.5	24.5–36.7	24.7–37.0
95	24.9–37.2	25.2–37.4	25.4–37.7	25.6–37.9	25.9–38.1
100	26.1–38.4	26.3–38.6	26.6–38.9	26.8–39.1	27.0–39.3
105	27.3–39.6	27.5–39.8	27.8–40.0	28.0–40.3	28.2–40.5
110	28.5–40.7	28.7–41.0	28.9–41.2	29.2–41.5	29.4–41.7
115	29.6–41.9	29.9–42.2	30.1–42.4	30.4–42.6	30.6–42.9

References:

Aperia A, Broberger O, Ekengren K, Wikstad I: Relationship between area and function of the kidney in well defined childhood nephropathies. Acta Radiol [Diagn] 1978; 19:186.

Currarino G: Roentgenographic estimation of kidney size in normal individuals with emphasis on children. AJR 1965; 93:464.

Eklöf O, Ringertz H: Kidney size in children. A method of assessment. Acta Radiol [Diagn] 1976a; 17:617.

Eklöf O, Ringertz H: Kidney size and growth in unilateral renal agenesis and in the remaining kidney following nephrectomy for Wilm's tumor. Acta Radiol [Diagn] 1976b; 17:601.

Jorulf H, Nordmark J, Jonsson A: Kidney size in infants and children assessed by area measurement. Acta Radiol [Diagn] 1978; 19:154.

Klare B, Geiselhardt B, Wesch H, Schärer K, Immich H, Willich E: Radiological kidney size in childhood. Pediatr Radiol 1980; 9:153.

UT2 Renal length, area and parenchymal thickness: ratio right/left kidney [radiography]

Referenced article:

Claësson I, Jacobsson B, Olsson T, Ringertz H: Assessment of renal parenchymal thickness in normal children. Acta Radiol [Diagn] 1981; 22:305.

Background:

See subsection UT1. Knowledge of renal right to left ratio is of value for screening purposes, as well as for follow-up of IVP evaluation.

Material:

Eklöf and Ringertz (1976) studied urographic AP films of 135 children, with an L1–L3 distance of 2.5–11.5 cm. All were normal.

Eklöf et al. (1976) studied urographic AP films of 142 children (106 girls and 36 boys). All had unilateral reduplication of the ureter on one side (61 right and 81 left) but were otherwise normal.

Method of assessment:

The renal length, area and parenchymal thickness were calculated as described in subsection UT1. The ratios were calculated by dividing the values on the right side with the values on the left (Table UT2.1).

Table UT2.1. Normal range ($-2SD$ to $+2SD$) for the ratio between right and left measure of renal length, area and upper and lower parenchymal thickness. (After Claësson et al. 1981)

Parameter	Ratio
Renal length	0.86–1.11
Renal area	0.74–1.19
Cranial pole parenchymal thickness	0.79–1.19
Caudal pole parenchymal thickness	0.80–1.23

References:

Eklöf O, Ringertz H: Kidney size in children. A method of assessment. Acta Radiol [Diagn] 1976; 17:617.

Eklöf O, Ringertz H, Tschäppeler H: Kidney size in children with unilateral urinary duplication. Acta Radiol [Diagn] 1976; 17:626.

UT3   Renal length/age [radiography]

Referenced article:

Curarrino G, Williams B, Dana K: Kidney length correlated with age: normal values in children. Radiology 1984; 150:703.

Background:

The most common and easily determined radiographic measure of renal size is length. It has been correlated with many different body parameters in children, of which age was the first (Hodson et al. 1962, 1975; Lebowitz et al. 1975). Age generally is a somewhat less accurate statistic but is easy to use.

Material:

Urograms of 262 children, aged 0–14.5 years were studied. All were interpreted as normal and 422 of the kidneys could be measured. No distinction was made between boys and girls or right and left kidney. The ethnic composition of the material was not stated. The focus–film distance was 100 cm.

Method of assessment:

The polar length of each kidney was measured independent of the long axis direction directly on the radiograph. Normal ranges are given in Table UT3.1.

Table UT3.1. Normal range (−2SD to +2SD) for renal length (cm) in children between 0.75 and 14.5 years of age. As an example a 6.75-year-old child has a 96% probability of having a renal length between 8.0 and 11.2 cm. (After Currarino et al. 1984)

Age (years)	−	+ 0.25	+ 0.50	+ 0.75
0	–	–	–	5.1– 8.2
1	5.2– 8.3	5.3– 8.5	5.5– 8.6	5.6– 8.8
2	5.8– 8.9	5.9– 9.0	6.0– 9.2	6.2– 9.3
3	6.3– 9.4	6.4– 9.5	6.5– 9.7	6.7– 9.8
4	6.8– 9.9	6.9–10.0	7.0–10.2	7.1–10.3
5	7.3–10.4	7.4–10.5	7.5–10.6	7.6–10.7
6	7.7–10.8	7.8–10.9	7.9–11.0	8.0–11.2
7	8.1–11.3	8.2–11.4	8.3–11.5	8.4–11.6
8	8.5–11.6	8.6–11.7	8.7–11.8	8.8–11.9
9	8.9–12.0	9.0–12.1	9.1–12.2	9.1–12.3
10	9.2–12.3	9.3–12.4	9.4–12.5	9.5–12.6
11	9.6–12.7	9.6–12.7	9.7–12.8	9.8–12.9
12	9.9–12.9	9.9–13.0	10.0–13.1	10.1–13.1
13	10.1–13.2	10.2–13.2	10.3–13.3	10.3–13.3
14	10.4–13.4	10.5–13.4	10.5–13.5	–

References:

Hodson CJ, Drewe JA, Karn MN, King A: Renal size in normal children. A radiographic study during life. Arch Dis Child 1962; 37:616.

Hodson CJ, Davies Z, Prescod A: Renal parenchymal radiographic measurement in infants and children. Pediatr Radiol 1975; 3:16.

Lebowitz RL, Hopkins T, Colodny AH: Measuring the kidneys. Practical applications using a growth and hypertrophy chart. Pediatr Radiol 1975; 4:37.

UT4   Renal length/age [ultrasound]

Referenced article:

Rosenbaum DM, Korngold E, Littlewood-Teele R: Sonographic assessment of renal length in normal children. AJR 1984; 142:467.

Background:

Ultrasound is today the primary modality in screening the kidneys of children with renal problems. The length of the kidney is the easiest parameter to assess, but volume has a more accurate correlation with most body size parameters in normal subjects (Han and Babcock 1985). There is no obvious 'internal' standard with sonography, such as the L1–L3 distance in radiography, even though attempts have been made to determine such parameters (Hederström 1985). Of 'external' parameters age has been used in a number of studies (Blaine et al. 1985; Dinkel et al. 1985, Han and Babcock 1985).

Material and method of assessment:

Sonograms from 203 patients, aged newborn to 19 years were studied. Patients with sonographic or clinical abnormalities of the urinary tract were excluded. No difference was made between right and left kidney or between sexes. The examinations were performed using a real-time sector scanner with 3.5–7.5 MHz transducers. The transducer was positioned to image the longest projection of the kidney. The length was measured on the films obtained (Table UT4.1).

Table UT4.1. Normal range (−2SD to +2SD) for sonographically determined renal length (cm) in children between 0 and 15.75 years of age. As an example a 6.75-year-old child has a 96% probability of having a renal length between 7.1 and 9.8 cm. (After Rosenbaum et al. 1984)

Age (years)	–	+ 0.25	+ 0.50	+ 0.75
0	3.8– 5.8	4.5– 6.6	4.7– 6.9	4.9– 7.1
1	5.1– 7.3	5.2– 7.5	5.4– 7.7	5.5– 7.8
2	5.6– 8.0	5.7– 8.1	5.8– 8.2	5.9– 8.4
3	6.0– 8.5	6.1– 8.6	6.2– 8.7	6.3– 8.8
4	6.4– 8.9	6.4– 9.0	6.5– 9.1	6.6– 9.2
5	6.7– 9.2	6.7– 9.3	6.8– 9.4	6.9– 9.5
6	6.9– 9.6	7.0– 9.6	7.0– 9.7	7.1– 9.8
7	7.2– 9.9	7.2– 9.9	7.3–10.0	7.3–10.1
8	7.4–10.2	7.5–10.2	7.5–10.3	7.6–10.4
9	7.6–10.4	7.7–10.5	7.7–10.5	7.8–10.6
10	7.8–10.7	7.9–10.7	7.9–10.8	8.0–10.9
11	8.0–10.9	8.1–11.0	8.1–11.0	8.2–11.1
12	8.2–11.1	8.2–11.2	8.3–11.2	8.3–11.3
13	8.4–11.4	8.4–11.4	8.5–11.5	8.5–11.5
14	8.6–11.6	8.6–11.6	8.6–11.7	8.7–11.7
15	8.7–11.8	8.8–11.8	8.8–11.9	8.8–11.9

References

Blaine CE, Bookstein FL, DiPietro MA, Kelsch RC: Sonographic standards for normal infant kidney length. AJR 1985; 145:1289.

Dinkel E, Ertel M, Dittrich M, Peters H, Berres M, Schulte-Wisserman H: Kidney size in childhood. Sonographical growth charts for kidney length and volume. Pediatr Radiol 1985; 15:38.

Han BK, Babcock DS: Sonographic measurements and appearance of normal kidneys in children. AJR 1985; 145:611.

Hederström E: Renal size parameter. A sonographic method for measuring lumbar vertebral height in children. Acta Radiol [Diagn] 1985; 26:693.

UT5 Renal length in neonates [ultrasound]

Referenced article:

Holloway H, Jones TB, Robinson AE, Harpen MD, Wiseman HJ: Sonographic determination of renal volumes in normal neonates. Pediatr Radiol 1983; 13:212.

Background:

See subsection UT4.

Material:

Ultrasound examinations of 62 normal term neonates were performed within the first week of life, using a 5 MHz transducer.

Method of assessment:

The greatest renal length as obtained from longitudinal scans was measured.

The renal volumes including the pelvic and calyceal structures were determined with two methods. One method summed plane-parallel slice areas multiplied by the slice thickness. The other method used the ellipsoid formula: renal volume = the product of the three principal axes of the kidney and the ellipsoid factor $\pi/6$.

Normal ranges for renal length and volume are given in Table UT5.1.

Table UT5.1. Normal range ($-2SD$ to $+2SD$) for renal length and volume in normal term neonates during the first week of life. (After Holloway et al. 1983)

Group	Renal length (cm)	Renal volume (cm³)
All kidneys	3.4–5.0	5.7–14.3
Male neonates	3.3–5.1	6.7–14.4
Female neonates	3.5–4.9	5.2–13.0
Right kidney	3.4–4.9	5.6–13.5
Left kidney	3.4–5.1	6.1–14.5

UT6   Renal length/body weight in premature infants [ultrasound]

Referenced article:

Schlesinger AE, Hedlund GL, Pierson WP, Null DM: Normal standards for kidney length in premature infants: Determination with US. Radiology 1987; 164:127.

Background:

See subsection UT4. In the premature infant the exclusion of renal disease is best performed with an ultrasonic determination of renal size as changes in that parameter often precede other sonographic changes in the kidney.

Material:

Sonograms from 52 healthy but premature children within the first 3 days of life were used. The gestational age ranged from 23 to 37 weeks and the body weight from 0.53 to 3.68 kg. No difference between right and left kidney or between boys and girls was found. The measurements of the 104 kidneys were performed with a 5.5 MHz real-time sector scanner.

Method of assessment:

The largest longitudinal dimension of the kidney was measured (Table UT6.1).

Table UT6.1. Normal range (−2SD to +2SD) for renal length (cm) related to body weight for premature infants between the 23rd and 37th gestational week. As an example a premature but normal infant weighing 1.8 kg has a 96% probability of having kidneys that are between 3.54 and 4.47 cm long. (After Schlesinger et al. 1985)

Body weight (kg)		+ 0.1	+ 0.2	+ 0.3	+ 0.4
0.5	–	2.64–3.57	2.72–3.65	2.79–3.72	2.87–3.80
1.0	2.94–3.87	3.01–3.95	3.09–4.02	3.16–4.10	3.24–4.17
1.5	3.31–4.25	3.39–4.32	3.46–4.39	3.54–4.47	3.61–4.54
2.0	3.69–4.62	3.76–4.69	3.84–4.77	3.91–4.84	3.99–4.92
2.5	4.06–4.99	4.13–5.07	4.21–5.14	4.28–5.22	4.36–5.29
3.0	4.43–5.37	–	–	–	–

UT7 Renal volume/body weight [ultrasound]

Referenced article:

Dinkel E, Ertel M, Dittrich M, Peters H, Berres M, Schulte-Wissermann H: Kidney size in childhood. Sonographical growth charts for kidney length and volume. Pediatr Radiol 1985; 15:38.

Background:

See subection UT6.

For screening purposes assessment of renal length is often enough but at follow-up measurement of renal volume may be desirable.

Material:

Sonograms from 325 children, aged 3 days–16 years, with a body weight from 1.8 to 73.8 kg, were studied. Only children with clinical and sonographic normal findings were included. The ultrasound examination was performed with a 3.5 MHz real-time sector scanner.

Method of assessment:

The length and depth of the kidney were measured in a maximum longitudinal plane. The maximum width and a second depth measurement were done at 90° to the first determination. The average depth measurement was multiplied with the other two axes and the factor $\pi/6 = 0.523$ to assess the volume, according to the ellipsoid formula (Geirsson et al. 1982). Normal ranges of renal volume are given in Table UT7.1.

Table UT7.1. Normal range ($-2SD$ to $+2SD$) for renal volume (cm³) related to body weight in children between 2 and 54 kg. For example, a child weighing 38 kg has a 96% probability of having renal volumes of each kidney between 54 and 124 cm³. (After Dinkel et al. 1985)

Body weight (kg)		+ 1	+ 2	+ 3	+ 4
0			4–11	6–16	8–20
5	10–24	12–28	13–32	15–35	17–39
10	18–42	20–46	21–49	23–52	24–55
15	25–58	27–61	28–64	29–67	31–70
20	32–73	33–76	34–79	36–82	37–85
25	38–88	39–91	41–93	42–96	43–99
30	44–102	46–105	47–108	48–111	49–114
35	50–116	52–119	53–122	54–124	55–127
40	56–130	57–132	58–135	59–138	60–140
45	61–143	62–146	63–148	65–151	66–154
50	67–156	69–159	70–162	71–164	72–167

Reference:

Geirsson RT, Christie AD, Patel N: Ultrasound volume measurements comparing a prolate ellipsoid method with a parallel planimetric area method against a known volume. J Clin Ultrasound 1982; 10:329.

UT8 Renal echogenicity/age [ultrasound]

Referenced article:

Han BK, Babcock DS: Sonographic measurements and appearance of normal kidneys in children. AJR 1985; 145:611.

Background:

Renal echogenicity and renal sinus echoes change considerably during the first years of life. Standards for normal values according to age are therefore important.

Material:

Ultrasound examinations of the abdomen were performed in 122 normal children, aged newborn–17 years. The examinations were performed with a mechanical sector scanner, using 3.5–7.5 MHz transducers.

Methods of assessment:

The echogenicity of the renal cortical parenchyma of the right kidney was compared with that of the liver and the echogenicity of the left kidney with the spleen. The medullary pyramids were assessed as prominent or not and the central renal sinus echoes were classified according to the following scale: same as the cortex, slightly echogenic, moderately echogenic, or high intensity echoes, as seen in adults.

The percentage occurrence of the different aspects of echogenicity are given in Table UT8.1.

Table UT8.1. The percentage occurrence of different aspects of renal echogenicity in children at different ages. (After Han and Babcock 1985)

	Percentage occurrence					
	Newborn	1–6 m	7–11 m	1–3 y	4–9 y	> 10 y
Right kidney less echogenic than liver	35	85	89	83	100	100
Left kidney less echogenic than spleen	50	92	100	100	100	100
Pyramids prominent	100	62	11	0	0	0
Central sinus echoes:						
Equal to parenchyma	25	0	0	0	0	0
Slightly echogenic	75	50	22	0	0	0
Moderately echogenic	0	50	78	67	30	9
Marked echogenic as in adults	0	0	0	33	70	91

UT9 Skin-to-kidney distance/weight [CT (scintigraphy)]

Referenced article:

Maneval DC, Magill HL, Cypess AM, Rodman JH: Measurement of skin-to-kidney distance in children: implications for quantitative renography. J Nucl Med 1990; 31:287.

Background:

Knowledge of the skin-to-kidney centre distance is important for quantification of renal function using a gamma camera. If interindividual variations in this distance are not recognised, significant errors in quantitative pediatric renography may result (Gordon et al. 1987).

Material:

CT examinations of the abdomen were performed in 60 patients, 10–70 kg of weight. The slice thickness was 8 mm and a majority had had low osmolality contrast medium intravenously to enhance visualisation.

Method of assessment:

Renal depth was determined by identifying the midtransverse section of each kidney. At this level the perpendicular distance from the dorsal skin surface to the kidney centre was measured. The results are summarised in Table UT9.1.

Table UT9.1. Normal range (−2SD to +2SD) of skin-to-kidney centre distance (cm) for both sexes given for body weight between 10 and 70 kg. Example: a normal child weighing 57 kg has a 96% probability of having a skin-to-kidney centre distance between 5.4 and 7.7 cm. (After Maneval et al. 1990)

Body weight (kg)	+ 1	+ 2	+ 3	+ 4
10	1.9–4.2	2.0–4.3	2.0–4.3	2.1–4.4	2.2–4.5
15	2.3–4.6	2.3–4.6	2.4–4.7	2.5–4.8	2.6–4.9
20	2.6–4.9	2.7–5.0	2.8–5.1	2.9–5.2	2.9–5.2
25	3.0–5.3	3.1–5.4	3.2–5.5	3.2–5.5	3.3–5.6
30	3.4–5.7	3.5–5.8	3.5–5.8	3.6–5.9	3.7–6.0
35	3.7–6.0	3.8–6.1	3.9–6.2	4.0–6.3	4.0–6.3
40	4.1–6.4	4.2–6.5	4.3–6.6	4.3–6.6	4.4–6.7
45	4.5–6.8	4.6–6.9	4.6–6.9	4.7–7.0	4.8–7.1
50	4.9–7.2	4.9–7.2	5.0–7.3	5.1–7.4	5.2–7.5
55	5.2–7.5	5.3–7.6	5.4–7.7	5.5–7.8	5.5–7.8
60	5.6–7.9	5.7–8.0	5.8–8.1	5.8–8.1	5.9–8.2
65	6.0–8.3	6.0–8.3	6.1–8.4	6.2–8.5	6.3–8.6
70	6.3–8.6	6.4–8.7	6.5–8.8	6.6–8.9	6.6–8.9

Reference:

Gordon I, Evans K, Peters AM, Kelly J, Morales BN, Goldraich N, Yau A: The quantitation of ^{99m}Tc–DMSA in paediatrics. Nucl Med Commun 1987; 8:661.

UT10   Ureteral submucosal tunnel length/height [ultrasound]
Ureteral submucosal tunnel length/age [ultrasound]

Referenced article:

Marchal GJ, Baert AL, Eeckels R, Proesmans W: Sonographic evaluation of the normal ureteral submucosal tunnel in infancy and childhood. Pediatr Radiol 1983; 13:125.

Background:

The anatomy of the ureterovesical junction is of importance for the evaluation of the refluxing ureter in children. Using the filled bladder as an acoustic window both the extra- and intravesical part of the ureter can be assessed. The submucosal ureteral segment is the part that runs parallel to the bladder wall, between the transmural ureteral segment and the meatus (Figure UT10.1). It is abnormally short or absent in refluxing ureters.

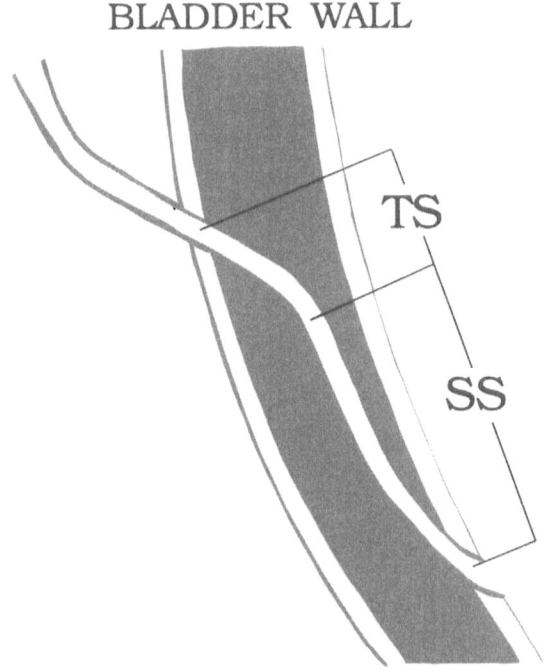

Figure UT10.1. The intramural part of the distal ureter. TS, transmural segment; SS, submucosal segment, used for the present measurements. (After Marchal et al. 1983.)

Table UT10.1. Lower normal limits (−2SD) for the ureteral submucosal tunnel length (cm) for children with height between 100 and 189 cm. As an example a 133 cm tall normal child has a 98% probability of having a ureteral submucosal tunnel on ultrasound that is 0.62 cm or longer. (After Marchal et al. 1983)

Height (cm)	0	+1	+2	+3	+4	+5	+6	+7	+8	+9
100	0.29	0.30	0.31	0.32	0.33	0.34	0.35	0.36	0.37	0.38
110	0.39	0.40	0.41	0.42	0.43	0.44	0.45	0.46	0.47	0.48
120	0.49	0.50	0.51	0.52	0.53	0.54	0.55	0.56	0.57	0.58
130	0.59	0.60	0.61	0.62	0.63	0.64	0.65	0.66	0.67	0.68
140	0.69	0.70	0.71	0.72	0.73	0.74	0.75	0.76	0.77	0.78
150	0.79	0.80	0.81	0.81	0.82	0.83	0.84	0.85	0.86	0.87
160	0.88	0.89	0.90	0.91	0.92	0.93	0.94	0.95	0.96	0.97
170	0.98	0.99	1.00	1.01	1.01	1.02	1.03	10.4	10.5	1.06
180	1.07	1.08	1.09	1.10	1.11	1.12	1.13	1.14	1.15	1.15

Material:

Ultrasound examinations in 35 normal children and young adults from 3 years of age, with even sex distribution were studied. A total of 58 ureters could be evaluated. A sector scanner with a 5.0 MHz transducer was used. Technical limitations made the assessments unapplicable in neonates and infants.

Method of assessment:

The visualisation of the distal ureter was optimal when both the extra- and intravesical part could be seen in the same plane. The submucosal part of the latter was measured where it ran parallel to the bladder wall. The measurement wsa taken between the meatus and the point where the ureter turns away from the inner bladder surface in its transmural part (Figure UT10.1). The results are summarised in Tables UT10.1 and UT10.2.

Table UT10.2. Lower limit for the ureteral submucosal tunnel length (cm) for children between 3 and 17 years of age. As an example a 10-year-old child should have a ureteral submucosal tunnel length below 0.85 cm. (After Marchal et al. 1983)

Age (years)	Tunnel length (cm)	Age (years)	Tunnel length (cm)	Age (years)	Tunnel length (cm)
3	0.61	4	0.64	5	0.68
6	0.71	7	0.74	8	0.78
9	0.81	10	0.85	11	0.88
12	0.91	13	0.95	14	0.98
15	1.01	16	1.05	17	1.08

UT11 Ureteral diameter/L1–L3 [radiography]
Ureteral diameter/age [radiography]

Referenced article:

Hellström M, Hjelmås K, Jacobson B, Jodal U, Odén A: Normal ureteral diameter in infancy and childhood. Acta Radiol [Diagn] 1985; 26:433.

Background:

An evaluation of the upper urinary tract in children always includes the width of the ureters as well as possible distension of the renal pelvis and calyces. Any effective measure to assess if the widest part of the ureter is abnormally dilated must include a body reference such as age or, for conformity with other methods, the L1–L3 distance.

Material:

Urograms from 194 children, aged 0–16 years were studied. The sex distribution was even. All children were considered normal and 330 ureters were included in the study. An IVP was performed using 4 ml/kg of contrast medium up to 5 kg body weight, 20 ml between 5 and 10 kg, 30 ml between 10 and 20 kg, and 40 ml in children over 20 kg. The IVP films were exposed in either the supine or prone position with a film–focus distance of 100 cm and a table top–film distance of 10 cm. Only films obtained without abdominal compression and ureters visualised for half or more of their total length on at least one IVP film were accepted. The ureteral visualisation was defined as the added length of the ureteral contrast medium filled segments in relation to the total length of the ureter.

Method of measurement:

The widest diameter of the ureter was measured avoiding the juxtapelvic cone-shaped part of the ureter. The right ureter was statistically significantly wider than the left, on average 0.06 cm. No correction for magnification, sex or body position was applied. The results are summarised in Tables UT11.1 and UT11.2.

Table UT11.1. Upper normal (+2SD) limits for ureteral diameter (cm) measured at its widest point, in children up to 16 years, related to the length of the lumbar segment L1–L3 including the intervertebral spaces. For example, a normal child with L1–L3 = 8.3 cm has a 98% probability of having a ureteral diameter equal to or below 0.78 cm. (After Hellström et al. 1985)

L1–L3 (cm)	–	+ 0.1	+ 0.2	+ 0.3	+ 0.4	+ 0.5	+ 0.6	+ 0.7	+ 0.8	+ 0.9
3	0.46	0.46	0.47	0.47	0.48	0.48	0.49	0.49	0.50	0.50
4	0.51	0.51	0.52	0.52	0.52	0.54	0.54	0.55	0.55	0.56
5	0.56	0.57	0.57	0.58	0.59	0.59	0.60	0.60	0.61	0.62
6	0.62	0.63	0.64	0.64	0.65	0.66	0.66	0.67	0.67	0.68
7	0.69	0.70	0.70	0.71	0.72	0.72	0.73	0.74	0.74	0.75
8	0.76	0.77	0.77	0.78	0.79	0.80	0.80	0.81	0.82	0.83
9	0.83	0.84	0.85	0.86	0.86	0.87	0.88	0.89	0.90	0.91
10	0.91	0.92	0.93	0.94	0.95	0.96	0.96	0.97	0.98	0.99
11	1.00	1.01	1.02	1.02	1.03	1.04	1.05	1.06	1.07	1.08

Table UT11.2. Upper normal (+2SD) limits for ureteral diamter (cm) in children up to 16 years related to age. As an example a normal 8.25-year-old child has a 98% probability of having ureteral diameter equal to or below 0.79 cm. (After Hellström et al. 1985)

Age (years)	–	+ 0.25	+ 0.50	+ 0.75
0	0.51	0.52	0.53	0.54
1	0.54	0.55	0.56	0.57
2	0.58	0.59	0.60	0.60
3	0.61	0.62	0.63	0.64
4	0.65	0.66	0.66	0.67
5	0.68	0.69	0.70	0.71
6	0.71	0.72	0.73	0.74
7	0.75	0.75	0.76	0.77
8	0.78	0.79	0.79	0.80
9	0.81	0.82	0.83	0.83
10	0.84	0.85	0.86	0.87
11	0.87	0.88	0.89	0.90
12	0.90	0.91	0.92	0.93
13	0.93	0.94	0.95	0.96
14	0.96	0.97	0.98	0.99
15	0.99	1.00	1.01	1.02

UT12 Bladder capacity/L1–L3 [radiography]
Bladder proportions [radiography]

Referenced article:

Engström CF, Ringertz H: Radiologic method to assess urinary bladder capacity and proportions in children. Acta Radiol [Diagn] 1984; 25:33.

Background:

Bladder capacity can be of importance in pediatric urology both when the bladder is too small, most commonly in enuresis (Ringertz 1984), or too large. Bladder capacity can be established as infused volume at a given pressure. It may also be estimated radiologically, at micturition urethrocystography (MUC) using radiography, scintigraphy or ultrasound. The determination ought, however, to be performed under controlled pressure conditions, normally at bladder catheterisation. The referenced article presents a method that uses the bladder capacity assessed either from the amount of contrast medium infused or from the measurements of the bladder from AP and lateral MUC films.

Material:

MUC examinations were carried out in 97 girls and 42 boys between 0 and 15 years of age, examined 4–8 weeks after a urinary tract infection. All had normal radiological and clinical findings.

Method of assessment:

The bladder capacity was defined during bladder catheterisation as the amount of infused fluid after bladder emptying or from radiographic films of the bladder in AP and lateral projection at early voiding during MUC. The capacity

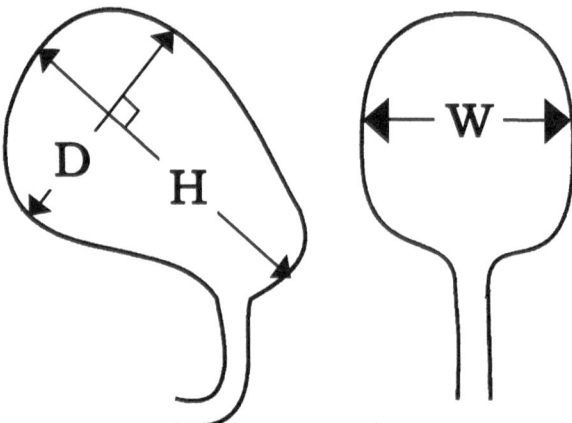

Figure UT12.1. Diameters used for calculation of bladder capacity. (After Engström and Ringertz 1984.)

Table UT12.1. Normal range (−2SD to +2SD) for the diameter product of the bladder related to the length of the lumbar segment L1–L3 including the intervertebral spaces. As an example a child with L1–L3 = 7.3 cm has a 96% probability of having a diameter product between 224 and 591 ml at 50 cm of contrast media pressure. (After Engström and Ringertz 1984)

L1–L3 (cm)	−	+ 0.1	+ 0.2	+ 0.3	+ 0.4
3.0	33–88	36–94	38–101	41–108	44–115
3.5	46–122	49–130	52–138	55–146	58–154
4.0	62–163	65–172	68–181	72–190	76–200
4.5	79–210	83–220	87–230	91–241	95–252
5.0	99–263	104–274	108–286	113–298	117–310
5.5	122–322	127–335	132–348	137–361	142–375
6.0	147–388	152–402	158–417	163–431	169–446
6.5	174–461	180–476	186–492	192–508	198–524
7.0	204–541	211–557	217–574	224–591	230–609
7.5	237–627	244–645	251–663	258–682	265–700
8.0	272–720	280–739	287–759	295–779	302–799
8.5	310–819	318–840	326–861	334–883	342–904
9.0	350–926	359–948	367–971	376–994	385–1017
9.5	393–1040	402–1064	411–1087	421–1112	430–1136
10.0	439–1161	449–1186	458–1211	468–1237	478–1263
10.5	488–1289	498–1315	508–1342	518–1369	528–1396
11.0	539–1424	549–1452	560–1480	571–1508	582–1537

assessed corresponded to the pressure of the infused fluid using a level of the infusion filter 50 cm above the estimated level of the centre of the bladder (Koff et al. 1979).

The bladder capacity as calculated from the MUC films assumes a film–focus distance of 110 cm and table top to film distance of 10 cm. The distance from the bladder to the film varies with bladder size and is included in the calculations leading to values given in Table UT12.1. The width (W) is measured on the AP film and the height (H) and depth (D) on the lateral film. The height is measured as the longest distance more or less parallel to the sacrum, the depth at right angles to the height (Figure UT12.1).

The diameter product W × H × D is entered into Table UT12.1. This value is related to the L1–L3 distance including the intervertebral spaces as measured from the lumbar spine in the frontal projection.

References:

Koff SA, Fischer CP, Poznanski AK: Cystourethrography. The effect of reservoir height upon intravesical pressure. Pediatr Radiol 1979; 8:21.
Ringertz H: Bladder capacity, urethral sensation and lumbosacral anomalies in children with enuresis. Acta Radiol [Diagn] 1984; 25:45.

UT13 Bladder wall thickness [ultrasound]

Referenced article:

Jequier S, Rousseau O: Sonographic measurements of the normal bladder wall in children. AJR 1987; 149:563.

Background:

The bladder wall thickness is influenced by a number of infectious, inflammatory, and toxic states. Using ultrasonography the wall is easily defined.

Material:

Ultrasound examinations of the bladder were performed in 410 children of either sex examined for non-urinary tract causes and found to have a normal urinary tract. Real-time transducers of 5 or 7.5 MHz were used.

Method of assessment:

The thickness of the bladder wall was measured posterolateral to the trigone of the bladder. At the same time the bladder volume was assessed as empty, half full, full or distended. This corresponded roughly to calculated values of: less than 10%, between 10% and 25%, between 25% and 90%, and more than 90% of maximal capacity, respectively. The results are summarised in Table UT13.1.

Table UT13.1. Normal range ($-2SD$ to $+2SD$) of bladder wall thickness according to fullness of the bladder. No statistical variation with age or sex was demonstrated. (After Jequier and Rousseau 1987)

Status	% of capacity	Bladder wall thickness (cm)
Empty bladder	0–10	0.16–0.39
Half full bladder	10–25	0.15–0.27
Full bladder	25–90	0.11–0.27
Distended bladder	90–100	0.04–0.27

UT14 Adrenal size/age: newborn [ultrasound]

Referenced article:

Scott EM, Thomas A, McGarrigle HHG, Lachelin GCL: Serial adrenal ultrasonography in normal neonates. J Ultrasound 1990; 9:279.

Background:

During the first weeks of life, the fetal zone of the adrenal cortex is subject to marked involution, and at the same time, there is proliferation of the definitive zone. Standards for the normal changes in size and appearance of the adrenal gland during the first weeks of life are therefore valuable.

Material:

Serial adrenal ultrasound examinations were performed on each of 12 healthy term infants on days 1, 3, 5, 11, 21 and 42, using a high-resolution real-time computerised phased array sector scanner with a 5 MHz transducer. The right adrenal was viewed with the child in the supine position, using the liver as an acoustic window; the left adrenal was visualised with the body in the right lateral decubitus position using the spleen as an acoustic window. Having obtained a longitudinal view of the kidney, the transverse view of the kidney was obtained by rotating the transducer through 90°. The adrenal was seen in transverse section by identifying the upper pole of the kidney and then angling the transducer slightly. The longitudinal views of the adrenal were obtained by visualising the kidney longitudinally and then angling the transducer about 30° medially.

Method of assessment:

The AP and transverse diameters were measured in the transverse section of the adrenal gland; the longitudinal diameter was measured in the longitudinal view (Figure UT14.1). The results are summarised in Table UT14.1.

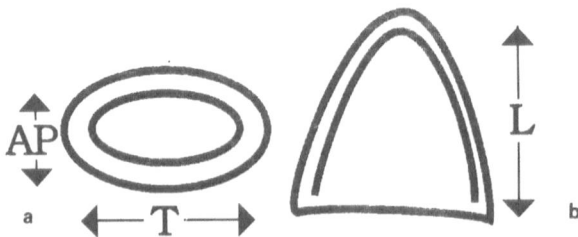

Figure UT14.1. Diameters of the adrenal gland. **a** Transverse section: AP, AP diameter; T, transverse diameter. **b** Longitudinal view: L, Longitudinal diameter. (After Scott et al. 1990.)

Table UT14.1. Normal range (−2SD to +2SD) for ultrasonographically determined adrenal diameters in the normal newborn. Values are given for neonates from 1 day to 6 weeks of age. (After Scott et al. 1990)

Age (days)	Adrenal diameters (mm)		
	Transverse	AP	Length
1	10.4–22.0	4.1–12.3	9.1–19.9
2	10.0–21.2	4.1–11.9	8.7–19.0
3	9.7–20.6	4.1–11.5	8.5–18.3
4	9.5–20.1	4.0–11.2	8.2–17.7
5	9.3–19.6	4.0–10.9	8.0–17.2
6	9.1–19.2	4.0–10.7	7.8–16.7
7	8.9–18.9	4.0–10.5	7.6–16.3
14	8.0–16.8	3.9– 9.2	6.7–13.8
21	7.2–15.2	3.8– 8.2	5.9–12.0
28	6.6–13.8	3.8– 7.4	5.3–10.4
35	6.0–12.6	3.7– 6.7	4.7– 9.1
42	5.6–11.5	3.7– 6.1	4.2– 7.8

Appendices

Appendix I. Nomogram for calculation of body surface area

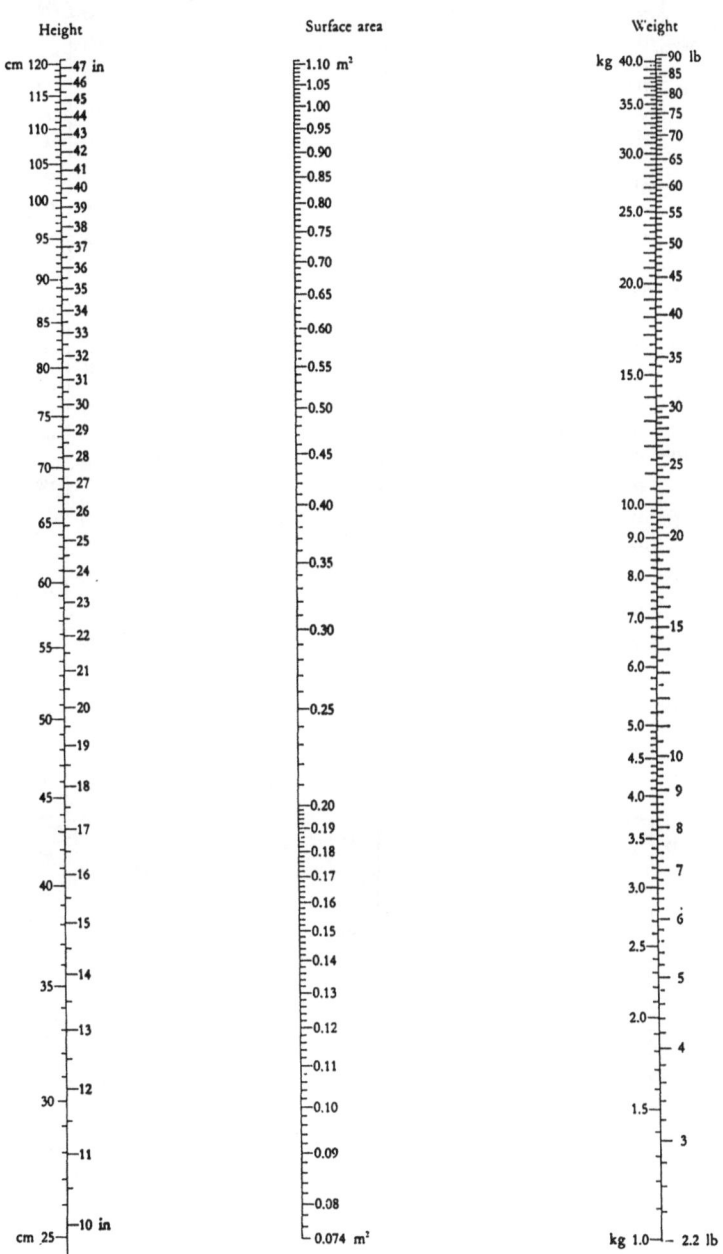

Nomogram according to Du Bois and Du Bois (1916). (*Continued on next page*)

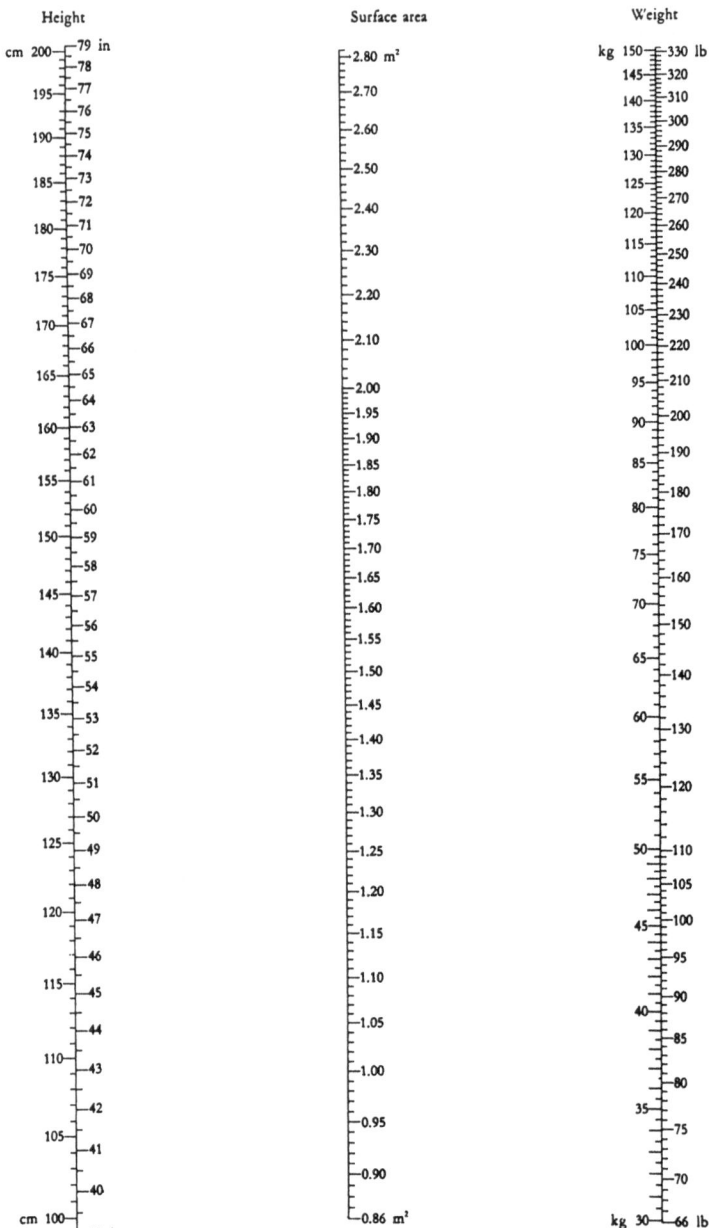

Nomogram according to Du Bois and Du Bois (1916). (*Continued*)

Appendix II.   Statistical considerations

Normal values and other numeric information useful for measurements in radiology are published in a multitude of ways. Results are often reported in the form or more or less complex equations which in most cases prohibit the proper routine use of the information. In addition, mean and standard deviation (SD) are used in different ways by different authors. This is especially true for linear and curvilinear regressions with different types of standard error of the estimate (SEE).

We have tried to present the results in the referenced articles in as standardised a way as possible. The normal range has been defined as tolerance limits for −2SD to +2SD. We have simplified this range to 96% probability and, in the cases when only the upper or lower normal limit is available or meaningful, as 98%.

When equations were given in the referenced papers, they have normally been used. This is true whether SD or SEE were stated or not. If normal limits were given in illustrations without reference to equations, we have used magnification and computerised analyses of the published line or curve to determine a useful equation. The error introduced in this way has been negligible compared with such factors as thickness of the lines in the original drawing etc.

Tables of means and SD related to age, body weight, height, body surface area, etc. have been plotted graphically. If linear or reasonable curvilinear conditions apply to the upper and lower normal limit values the best fit equation has been calculated for each limit. The correlation for these 'best fits' has always been significant and the coefficient of correlation better than 0.8. In some instances, when no significant change with age, body weight, etc. could be demonstrated, the material has been summarised as one normal range. When a significant change was seen but no reasonable curve fit for the observed limit the varying normal ranges have been used.

In some instances different regression equations and tolerance limits for different ranges were given in the referenced articles. The limits have then been plotted and smoothing of the transition between the two ranges has been applied to avoid abrupt changes of the normal range leading to artifacts in clinical longitudinal applications for the individual patient.

Some of the above described techniques are unorthodox and introduce possible errors. We have assessed them as acceptable considering the consequences of not using them, especially as the present book is primarily aimed at use in normal practical working conditions, in the routine clinical setting.

The calculations made have been computerised and all equations used have been introduced in computer programs to produce the tables. The values for the measurements have in most instances been given with one decimal more than normal precision of the technique used. Thus, the observed value can be assessed more easily as within or outside the normal range.

A more detailed description of the statistical and mathematical approach for all the tables is given below.

Section	Table	Method
SK1	SK1.1	Primary data available
	SK1.2	Primary data available
SK2	SK2.1	Recalculation of given data from 90% to 96% probability from tables of normal distributions. Smoothed transition at 3 years
SK3	SK3.1	Visual estimate of data, recalculation from 90% to 96% probability from tables of normal distributions. Smoothed transition at 2 years
SK4	SK4.1	Linear equations of + and − 2SD calculated from figure
SK5	SK5.1	Recalculation of given data from 80% to 96% probability from tables of normal distributions
SK6	SK6.1	Calculations from table of individual values
SK7	SK7.1	Values given in referenced article
SK8	SK8.1	Best fit linear equations calculated for each − and + 2SD set of data from given tables
	SK8.2	Same as SK8.1
SK9	SK9.1	Best fit linear equations calculated for sets of − and + 2SD values calculated from given tables
	SK9.2	Normal range for each age calculated from table values of mean and SD. No significant trend with age observed
SP1	SP1.1	No data available to calculate normal range except above 2 years of age. Mean values and range from text and figure of referenced article
SP2	SP2.1	Range calculated from values given in table of referenced article
	SP2.2	Only mean values available
SP3	SP3.1	Ranges calculated from individual values given in the referenced article
SP4	SP4.1	Best fit linear equations calculated for sets of − and + 2SD values calculated from given tables
SP5	SP5.1	Best fit linear equations calculated for sets of mean values for both sexes combined, as given in the referenced article. Average SDs calculated from given values and applied
SP6	SP6.1	Ranges calculated from mean and SD values given in table in the referenced article
	SP6.2	Best fit 'square root of age' equations calculated for sets of − and + 2SD values calculated from mean and SD values given in table
SP7	SP7.1	Linear equation given. SD assessed from figure
SP8	SP8.1	All parameters of linear equations given in referenced article
SP9	SP9.1	Ranges for each level calculated from given mean and SD values

Section	Table	Method
	SP9.2	Ranges for each level calculated from given values
SP10	SP10.1	Ranges taken from table in referenced article
PH1	PH1.1	Ranges given in table of referenced article
PH2	PH2.1	Best fit 'square root of age' equations calculated for sets of − and + 2 SD values calculated from values given in a table in the first referenced article and calculated from given data in the other
PH3	PH3.1	Upper value for normal range given in referenced article
PH4	PH4.1	Smoothed values from extreme range in figure of second referenced article
	PH4.2	Best fit linear equations calculated from given − and + 2SD values calculated from table values of mean and SD in the third referenced article
PH5	PH5.1	Smoothed values from extreme range in figure of the referenced article
PH6	PH6.1	The linear equations given in the referenced article were used. As no significant difference between sex was seen the extreme value was used to get a common table. Thus −2SD for boys and +2SD for girls was used
	PH6.2	The exponential equations given were used
PH7	PH7.1	Best fit linear equations calculated from given − and + 2SD values calculated from table values of mean and SD in the second referenced article
EX1	EX1.1	The published linear equations with standard error were used
	EX1.2	The published linear equations with standard error were used
EX2	EX2.1	Values calculated from mean and SD values given
EX3	EX3.1	Best fit 'square root of age' equations calculated for sets of − and + 2SD values calculated from mean and SD values given in a table in the referenced article
EX4	EX4.1	Values as published
EX5	EX5.1	Linear equations for normal ranges assessed from figures in referenced article. Smoothing applied in the range for femoral metaphyseal width between 53 and 63 mm
	EX5.2	Linear equations for normal range assessed from figures in referenced article. Smoothing applied in the range for femoral epiphyseal width between 52 and 59 mm
EX6	EX6.1	Normal range calculated from values of mean and SD given in referenced article

Section	Table	Method
EX7	EX7.1	Normal ranges assessed from figures in the referenced article
EX8	EX8.1	Adapted from referenced article
EX9	EX9.1	Normal range calculated from values of mean and SD given in referenced article
EX10	EX10.1	For muscle thickness best fit 'square root of age' equations were calculated from raw values of mean and SD published in referenced article. For soft tissue thickness published logarithmic equations were used
BM1	BM1.1	Normal ranges calculated from mean and SD values given in referenced article
	BM1.2	Normal ranges calculated from mean and SD values given in referenced article
BM2	BM2.1	The linear equations for the normal ranges were assessed from figures in the referenced article
	BM2.2	The linear equations for the normal ranges were assessed from figures in the referenced article
BM3	BM3.1	Normal ranges calculated from mean and SD values given in referenced article
BM4	BM4.1	Best fit second degree equation was calculated from mean -2SD values given in table of the referenced article. Best fit linear equation was calculated from mean and $+2$SD values given
	BM4.2	Best fit second degree equation was calculated from mean -2SD values given in table of the referenced article. Best fit linear equation was calculated from mean and $+2$SD values given
BM5	BM5.1	Best fit linear equations calculated from given $-$ and $+2$SD values calculated from table values of mean and SD in the referenced article
RT1	RT1.1	Smoothed normal range from values calculated from mean and SD in table of referenced article
RT2	RT2.1	Normal ranges calculated from original distribution of observations given in the referenced article
RT3	RT3.1	Linear equations for normal range assessed from figure in the referenced article
RT4	RT4.1	Best fit linear equations calculated from given $-$ and $+2$SD values calculated from table values of mean. and SD in the referenced article
RT5	RT5.1	Normal ranges calculated from mean and SD values given in table of the referenced article
RT6	RT6.1	The normal range was calculated from the combined normal material of the referenced article using the mean and SD values given

Section	Table	Method
CV1	CV1.1	Primary data available
	CV1.2	Primary calculations available
	CV1.3	Normal range calculated from the regression equations, standard errors and correction factor equations of the referenced article
	CV1.4	Normal range calculated from the regression equations, standard errors and correction factor equations of the referenced article
	CV1.5	Normal range calculated from the regression equations, standard errors and correction factor equations of the referenced article
CV2	CV2.1	Normal range calculated from linear equations and SD given in the referenced article
CV3	CV3.1	Normal ranges given in table of referenced article
CV4	CV4.1	Normal range calculated from logarithmic equation given in referenced article
CV5	CV5.1	No significant difference between the four veins. Normal range for all together calculated from linear equations, correlation coefficients and standard errors of the estimate given in referenced article
CV6	CV6.1	Probabilities calculated from case distribution figure in the referenced article
CV7	CV7.1	Normal range calculated with linear equations and standard errors obtained from the individual observations as plotted in figures in the referenced article
AB1	AB1.1	Normal linear range assessed from the total distribution of the material in figure in the referenced article
	AB1.2	Normal range calculated with best fit 'square root of age' equations in turn calculated from mean and SD values in figure of referenced article
AB2	AB2.1	Normal range for liver volume calculated with linear equations assessed from figure in referenced article. Normal range for spleen volume calculated with linear equations in turn calculated from given regression equation and measured SD from figure
AB3	AB3.1	Normal range calculated with best fit linear equations in turn calculated from − and +2SD values calculated from mean and SD values of table in referenced article
AB4	AB4.1	Normal range calculated with best fit 'square root of age' equations in turn calculated from mean and SD values in figure of referenced article
	AB4.2	Extreme observed range has been used as an assessment of normal range due to limited number of observations

Section	Table	Method
AB5	AB5.1	Normal linear range calculated from regression equation and standard error assessed from the total distribution of the material in figure in the referenced article
AB6	AB6.1	Normal ranges calculated from one or more materials and the published mean, SD and number of observations of each material
AB7	AB7.1	Normal ranges calculated from mean and SD values of table in referenced article
AB8	AB8.1	Normal range calculated from best fit 'square root of age' equation with standard error both in turn calculated from given individual observations
AB9	AB9.1	Normal range calculated from distribution of observations in figure of referenced article
UT1	UT1.1	Normal range calculated from linear equations and standard error given in referenced article. Smoothing for values corresponding to L1–L3 38–57 mm
	UT1.2	Normal range calculated from linear equations and standard error given in referenced article. Smoothing for values corresponding to L1–L3 40–60 mm
	UT1.3	Normal ranges calculated from linear equations and standard error given in referenced article
UT2	UT2.1	Normal range calculated from mean and SD given in referenced article
UT3	UT3.1	Normal range calculated from second and third degree equations of regression and SD, respectively
UT4	UT4.1	Normal range calculated with best fit 'square root of age' equations calculated from mean and SD given in table of the referenced article
UT5	UT5.1	Normal ranges calculated from pooled data for right and left kidneys, mean and SD given in tables of referenced article
UT6	UT6.1	Normal range values adapted from table of referenced article
UT7	UT7.1	Normal range from logarithmic equation and lower limit for right and upper limit for left kidney as from figure in referenced article
UT8	UT8.1	Percentages obtained from figures of referenced article
UT9	UT9.1	Normal range calculated from given linear equation and assessment of SD from figure in the referenced article
UT10	UT10.1	Lower normal limits calculated from given linear equation and assessment of SD from figure in the referenced article

Section	Table	Method
	UT10.2	Lower normal limits calculated from given extreme limits in figure and table of the referenced article
UT11	UT11.1	Upper normal limits calculated with given equations for mean and standard error
	UT11.2	Upper normal limits calculated with given equations for mean and standard error
UT12	UT12.1	Normal range calculated from logarithmic equation and standard error as given in the referenced article
UT13	UT13.1	Normal ranges calculated from recalculation of mean and SD values given in table of the referenced article
UT14	UT14.1	Normal ranges calculated with best fit 'square root of age' equations calculated from mean and SD given in table of the referenced article